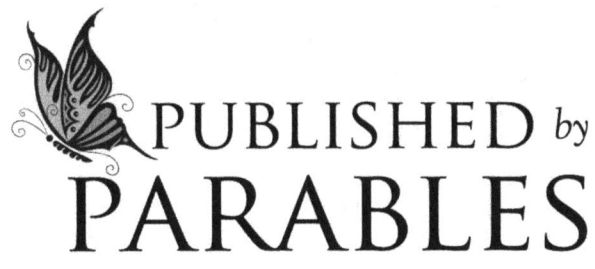

A Miracle Healing
Surviving Fungal Meningitis

Judy Arnold

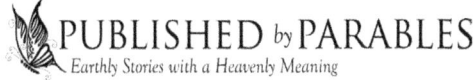

A Miracle Healing Surviving Fungal Meningitis
Judy Arnold

Copyright © Judy Arnold

Published By Parables
July, 2018

All Rights Reserved. No part of this book may be reproduced or utilized in any form or by any means, electronic or mechanical, including photocopying, recording, or by any information storage and retrieval system, without permission in writing from the author.

Unless otherwise specified Scripture quotations are taken from the authorized version of the King James Bible.

    ISBN 978-1-945698-64-4
    Printed in the United States of America

Readers should be aware that Internet Web sites offered as citations and/or sources for further information may have been changed or disappeared between the time this was written and when it is read.

A Miracle Healing
Surviving Fungal Meningitis

Judy Arnold

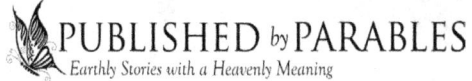
PUBLISHED by PARABLES
Earthly Stories with a Heavenly Meaning

This is a true story of one man's journey of surviving Fungal Meningitis. In spite of the circumstances that surrounds this deadly disease that only 10 out of 250 will survive. He is one of the few that escaped death to live a healthy life and tell many stories of Gods mercy, grace and love in a hopeless situation. Here is his story.

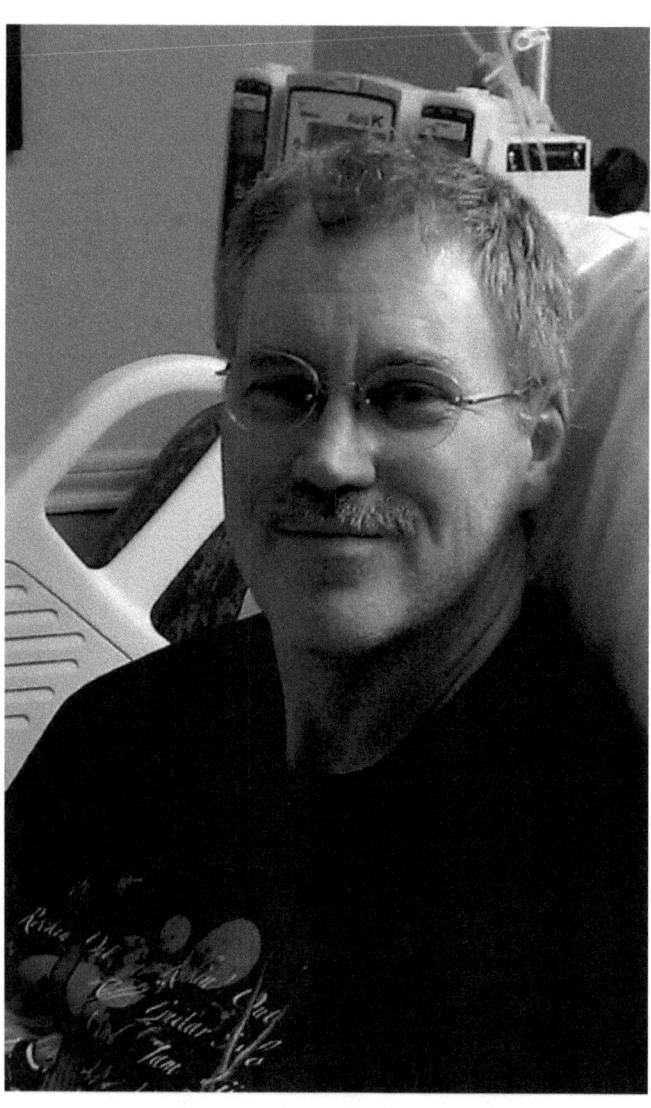

Dedication

This book is dedicated to God, our Father in heaven for his miracle working power! I also want to thank the awesome doctors and nurses at the NICU unit and the Neurology department 5th floor at Methodist hospital in Houston, Texas. Without your dedication, compassion and love for the patients that come under your care and their families, we wouldn't have survived our 32 day stay at Methodist hospital. All of you went out of your way, past your job duties to not only take care of my sick husband but made me feel like what I was going through mattered. The attention and help you showed both of us by getting us through such a difficult time will never be forgotten. We are grateful beyond words and thank you will never be enough. God bless you all!

Table of Contents

Dedication
Table of Contents 2
Chapter 1: The Onset 5
Chapter 2: Trusting Doctors 7
Chapter 3: Fear Creeps In 9
Chapter 4: A Hospital Nightmare 11
Chapter 5: Praying For Intervention 18
Chapter 6: The Ambulance Ride 21
Chapter 7: Emergency Room Chaos 23
Chapter 8: Unprofessional Behavior 26
Chapter 9: A Deep Breath 28
Chapter 10: Hope Shattered 30
Chapter 11: A Broken Vessel 33
Chapter 12: My Faith Tested 35
Chapter 13: A Sisters Love 38
Chapter 14: Looking Back 40
Chapter 15: An Unexpected Touch 42
Chapter 16: A Place to Stay 44
Chapter 17: God Speaks 46
Chapter 18 A Time of Stretching 48
Chapter 19: Pray Without Ceasing 51
Chapter 20: For the Love of God 53
Chapter 21: A Different Personality 56
Chapter 22: The New   Journey Begins 58
Chapter 23: House Building. Long Distance 61
Chapter 24: It's God or Nothing 63
Chapter 25 Curious Gary 66

Chapter 26: Visual Distortion	67
Chapter 27: The "Doctors" Diagnosis	69
Chapter 28: Corporate Prayer Honored	71
Chapter 29: Organ Shutdown	73
Chapter 30: Out of Immediate Danger	74
Chapter 31: Losing Track of Time	76
Chapter 32 Quiet Down Time	78
Chapter 33: Gary Reality Check	80
Chapter 34: A New Beginning	83
Chapter 35: Joyous News	85
Chapter 36: The Nurses	86
Chapter 37: 1000 Questions	89
Chapter 38: Faith and Determination	92
Chapter 39: Patience is a Virtue	94
Chapter 40: Memories Lost	96
Chapter 41: And He Walks	97
Chapter 42: A Beautiful Home Awaits	99
Chapter 43: The Final Lumbar Puncture	101
Chapter 44: Our New Goal-Home	103
Chapter 45: Angels Among Us	106
Chapter 46: Moving Day	108
Chapter 47: What Really Matters	110
Chapter 48: The Rest of the Story	112
Healing Scriptures	114
Faith Scriptures	115
Hope Scriptures	116
Love Scriptures	117

Judy Arnold

Chapter One
The Onset

Gary, being a strong healthy man at the age of 52, hadn't been to a doctor in over two years. So I wasn't concerned when he came home early from work during a normal day with a bad headache.

Not being the type of person for taking medication unless it is absolutely necessary or as a last resort, I was surprised when I offered him an Aleve and he gladly took it. I tried to get him to eat but all he wanted to do was shower and get in bed. Nothing ever kept him down so I wasn't too concerned.

He got up later that night in pain, took another Aleve and went back to bed. He was up bright and early the next day seemingly better so after breakfast he headed to work as usual. Around 2:30 pm that afternoon as I was busy cleaning house going through my daily routine when I heard his truck pull up.

I started to question why he was home early as he walked in but I could see the anguish on his face. Another headache, so bad this time he couldn't continue his work. He worked as a computer analyst and the pain made it impossible to stare at his computer any longer that day.

He was feeling bad pressure over his eyes so we both assumed it was sinus pressure from an infection. He took an over the counter sinus medication, ate supper, showered and was in bed by 8 pm. I was getting concerned at this point but he would have no part of going to the doctor. After two days in a row I was beginning to wonder what was going on. I'm not one to panic or overreact but this was just so unusual for him. I wasn't going to let it go on much longer even if I had to drag him kicking and screaming.

Chapter 2:
Trusting Doctors

We both assumed it was the onset of a bad sinus infection so we headed to a nearby urgent care hoping for some relief. I thought maybe he had a blockage in his sinus cavity which might be causing the severe headaches.

After waiting almost an hour we finally were able to see the doctor. A quick once over and we were headed home with a diagnosis of a sinus infection. He was given a steroid injection and a prescription of antibiotics. After getting it filled we headed home hoping for a better night.

Once again Gary was in bed by eight o' clock and I was getting a bit uneasy about this whole situation. A thousand things tend to race through your mind in situations like this but I tried not to worry for now.

The next morning he seemed somewhat better and went to work against my better judgement. Something just didn't seem right and that uneasiness was getting uncomfortable to me. He showed up again at noon with the worst headache yet.

He went to bed for a while but woke after a couple hours in so much pain that it didn't take any persuasion from me to go to the emergency room. After waiting for what seemed like an eternity, we were finally able to see a doctor. We discussed what had been going on for the last couple days and how concerned we both were about the severe headaches. Once again after only a 5 minute once over we had a diagnosis of a severe sinus infection.

I was beginning to question whether any of the doctors were competent. Were they so busy that they dismissed symptoms that were actually serious? Some things should have sent up red flags to the doctors and because it didn't it concerned me.

Another steroid shot, another round of antibiotics although he hadn't finished the ones from the prior doctor visit. We assumed the doctors knew what they were doing so we got the prescriptions and headed home.

It ended up being a horrible night for Gary and I was shocked when he got up for work the next day. I begged him to stay home but he was so worried about getting behind on his work. I cried and prayed after he left, scared of what was happening and not knowing what was to come. The next couple days we visited an emergency room in Lake Charles with same diagnosis.

Chapter 3:
Fear Creeps In

By 10 am Gary was home and in the worse pain I had ever seen for someone with a sinus infection. I had suffered with migraines for six years but never remember hurting like this and it scared me. He headed straight for the restroom and started to vomit. That was it, I called his regular family doctor to get him in that day.

After describing all the symptoms they of course wanted to see him as soon as possible. They scheduled an appointment for a couple hours later that afternoon. I was relieved because most of our family saw this doctor and I trusted him completely.

After the doctor examined Gary, he stated that if he had been treated twice for the same symptoms with no results then it obviously wasn't a sinus infection. After examining him concluded that it was possibly a migraine. Gary had never had a migraine before but we were grasping at straws to know what was wrong so we accepted his diagnosis. Gary was given a shot of Imitrex, a migraine medicine. He was instructed to lay down quietly in the room. We needed to stay and see if it worked before he would let us go home.

After about 20 minutes he seem to feel somewhat better although the headache wasn't completely gone. He was given a prescription for a second shot to be taken four hours later and we headed home.

Gary went straight to bed and slept for a while. I was relieved that he was feeling a little better and gave him the second shot when he woke up. But it was short lived. After only 30 minutes after the second shot, Gary was up vomiting worse than before.

I called the doctor terrified and he instructed us to go to ER and to tell the attending doctor to admit him for tests. Once again for the third time we were headed to a medical faculty seeking help.

After several tests were done, an IV was started to replenish his fluids. The doctor came in to tell us that all tests were negative and it was just a severe sinus infection.

I argued with the doctor about that diagnosis and told him our family physician had told us to come to ER and be admitted.

Evidently they hadn't received the orders and because of "protocols" they had no reason to keep him.

I begged him to keep him overnight for observation but he refused. For the life of me I couldn't imagine any doctor sending someone home in Gary's condition. Protocols or not, it seemed to me that more tests could have been ran. I got the feeling he just didn't want to take the extra step to help.

We headed home with still no answer and Gary sicker than he had been in the last five days.

Chapter 4: A Hospital Nightmare

Gary had a really bad night after leaving ER and I was on the phone to the doctor the next morning at eight am. As you can imagine our doctor was furious with the ER doctor and wasn't sure why they hadn't received the admission papers. Our doctor ordered a cat scan at the hospital and then sent paperwork so that everything would be in place when we got there.

We endured another long wait in admitting before we were taken back for the CAT scan. Afterwards we made our way back to ER. The paperwork was there and we were brought straight to a room after being admitted. I took a sigh of relief that at least we were finally in a place that they could find out what was wrong with my husband.

Day One
Nurses fluttered in and out doing vitals, drawing blood, starting an IV and asking more questions. Poor Gary tried to answer but was in too much pain and so very weak. After an hour or so, a nurse came in and gave him Demerol for pain. He was asleep in seconds and I was relieved for him. It was the first time in a week he had actually slept and didn't seem to be in pain.

Our family doctor visited around 6pm that day. I was happy to see him and bombarded him with questions. He had no idea what might be wrong but promised us he would get to the bottom of it. He mentioned doing a lumbar puncture but wanted to get the results of all the tests first.

The first day in the hospital ended without any results of what might be causing all of this. Gary was resting and out of pain for the moment and that was a blessing. I was relieved but tired and worried of what tomorrow would hold for us.

Day Two

As with day one, this morning started off with more tests to my weak sick husband. I felt so helpless and prayed continuously for God to help us find out what was wrong. He awoke this morning with the worse intense pain since the onset. As they injected more pain meds in his IV, I hoped we would get good news because the tests had to revel something besides a sinus infection.

Gary was getting progressively worse and I was scared to death that something really serious was wrong. I knew the tests were necessary but this was taking was too long and in my spirit I had an uneasy feeling that time was running out.

Today the vomiting stopped but he was weaker than the day before. He couldn't keep any food down, not even water.

I was getting angry at the lack of concern by the hospital staff. I asked several times a day if we had test results and when the doctor would be back in to see him. In my gut I knew this was turning into a life or death thing and it was about to get nasty around here.

Day Three

After three days the on call neurologist that was supposedly handling our case showed up. I always assumed if a doctor was "on call" and had a patient needing a neurological evaluation that he would see the patient the day they are admitted. But this was not the case and so I was already a little frustrated that as sick as Gary was that he had finally made an appearance.

As you can imagine, emotions were running high already and I tried my best to stay calm and patient. Gary was all that mattered at this point and I was just glad a specialist was going to assess him.

Nothing could have been further from the truth!

He was the least professional doctor I had ever encountered. His bedside manner was rude and he acted as if it was an inconvenience that he had to take his time to come by.

He plopped himself down on the couch, stretched out one leg and let his white coat fall open. I was in disbelief as he started asking Gary and I questions about what had happened. He acted more like he was there to watch a football game than assess a sick patient.

I was furious and it was hard to contain myself as I sat closed mouth until he finished his "opinion". That should have been a red flag to find another doctor but we were so desperate to get answers to this chaos so we listened quietly. He then asked about a knot Gary had on his forehead close to his scalp.

Gary explained that he had hit a corner of an open cabinet 20 years ago and that it was just a calcium deposit. Without even looking at Gary's chart or any of the tests results, he concluded that the cyst on his forehead was the culprit. Although Gary explained it had been there years and had never bothered him at all, his mind was made up. He scheduled an MRI of Gary's head to get a better look at the cyst.

I mentioned that his family doctor wanted to do a lumbar puncture but he shook his head and said it wasn't necessary. He muttered something about sending a neurosurgeon the next day to look at it. He acted like he didn't want it to be anything he would have to deal with.

I was dismayed and disappointed of the idea of another incompetent doctor and I knew at that moment we didn't want him to take care of Gary. I was so glad Gary's sister Crystal happened to be there to witness this irresponsible behavior and attitude from a doctor. She was just as upset as we were.

Red flag number two. These doctors were supposed to know What they were doing right?. I was beginning to question if we were at the right place to be helped. Another pain med injection, another night of restlessness and pain and not any closer to finding out what the hell was going on!!!

The next morning a neurosurgeon came in to see Gary and

looked at the bump on his scalp. He laughed and said there was no way that it was the cause of the headaches. He confirmed what we already knew so when the regular doctor came in later that morning, we advised him of what the neurosurgeon has said. He advised us to have the lumbar puncture but we told him the neurologist didn't want to do it. I also told him I was thinking about bringing Gary to Houston to a specialist. He agreed but informed us he was going to order the lumbar puncture himself. I was relieved because I felt like they would find something then.

That afternoon a guy from Gary's job came by to check on Gary and pray for him. As he sat on the side of the bed, we held hands and he began to pray. All of a sudden the door was literally kicked open and in came the neurologist. We all looked up startled as he began to raise his voice, almost screaming at us. He said our doctor had told him we wanted to go to Houston. He was furious and asked us why. As I started to explain, he cut me off and told us that if we weren't satisfied with his care we could find another doctor. I told him our doctor had ordered the lumbar puncture because we wanted to have it. In an elevated voice, he spouted "well good then, you can just stay with him because I will no longer treat him" and stormed out of the room.

Not once did he acknowledge or apologize for interrupting us while we were praying, I guess his pride was hurt but it was the most unprofessional display from a doctor I had ever seen. We apologized to our guest for his rude behavior and also informed our doctor what had happened. It was definitely time to find a new doctor and a better equipped hospital!

Day Four

As we patiently waited for the nurse to come get Gary for the lumbar puncture that was scheduled for nine am that morning, Gary became very agitated. At first I thought because the doctor had changed the pain medicine from Demerol to Dilaudid, a much stronger medication.

I wasn't sure what the side effects were but he was acting almost anxious.

I tried talking to him to keep him calm but he was thrashing around in the bed like he was hurting and frustrated. I was about to call the nurse when the tech showed up to take him down for the test.

It seemed like not any time had passed at all and they were wheeling him back in the room. I commented how little time it had taken but I was glad he was back. He seemed calm and it hit me as kind of strange. I ask him how the test went and he told me he didn't even feel the stick. I laughed and told him it was probably because of the pain med he has just had.

While he was gone, his first cousin Melanie had stopped by to check on him and was still there when he returned. After he settled down again he asked me when they were coming to get him for the lumbar puncture. I figured he was kind of confused from the pain meds so I leaned over and whispered that he had already finished the test. He looked bewildered at me and said I did?

Melanie talked to him a few minutes and as she was leaving he again asked her the same question. We looked at each other puzzled and again told him he was finished with the test. He seemed frustrated like he didn't believe us. Melanie left and said to call her if we needed anything.

A few minutes later Gary ask me again for the third time and then tried to sit up. I laid him back down and tried to tell him that he couldn't sit up for 12 hours after the lumbar puncture. I told him he could get a worse headache but it angered him. Once again he tried to get up and I began to feel like something was wrong.

The next thing that happened was so fast and unexpected it caught me off-guard. Within seconds Gary went from agitated to acting like a crazy person. I know that sounds cruel but I don't know any other way to describe it. He grabbed the handrails and sat up in bed abruptly.

I put my hands gently on his chest and tried to lay him back down but that was a mistake. As I looked in his face trying to talk to him, his eyes glassed over and he looked at me and started screaming "who are you and where am I?" The next thing I knew, he had grabbed me by my arms and shoved me so hard I fell on the couch next to the bed! I jumped up and pushed the nurses button screaming somebody help me now! I didn't realize how loud I was screaming because I was trying to scream over him. A male nurse coming down the hall had heard the commotion and ran in the room.

He pushed Gary down on the bed while calling for help and within seconds there were a room full of nurses. For being as weak as he was, his strength was unbelievable. He was kicking and screaming at the top of his lungs as they whisk me out of the room.

As I stood outside the room crying and scared to death, more nurses came and within seconds the room was filled with over 10 people. They gave him a narcotic to knock him out but it didn't work .As they struggled to hold him down, they gave him a second dose. A nurse brought me to the other end of the hall but I could still hear him screaming. All I remember was covering my ears and crying like a baby.

I was beside myself, terrified about what had just happened and not understanding any of it. All I knew was that something was severely wrong with Gary and if we didn't find out what that was, I was afraid he might not make it much longer. I called my oldest son, Ryan that was working just a mile from the hospital. I was hysterical and told him to come to the hospital because I thought his dad was dying. He was there in a matter of minutes and I was waiting by the elevator when it opened.

He was pale and I threw my arms around him sobbing. Gary was still screaming and Ryan asked me what had happened. I explained how Gary had went crazy then he went into the room hoping to see his dad. Seconds later he came out and said no one was allowed in there for now. A few minutes later the screaming finally stopped and a stream of nurses spilled out into the hallway.

One nurse was covered in blood and I started to panic. When she saw the look on my face, she quickly touched my arm to assure me everything was ok. In all the thrashing around and fighting, Gary had pulled his IV out. They ended up giving him three sedatives before he finally calmed down. Ryan was shook up and I was glad when his cousin Randy showed up. They went down the hall to talk. The elevator opened again and it was Ronnie, Gary's first cousin. They had been like brothers their whole life and I was glad to see him. He hugged me and I fell apart sobbing like a baby. He stuck his head in the room but Gary was out so I promised I would tell Gary he had stopped by.

Within minutes the nurse came out to inform me that they were taking Gary to ICU. When I went back into the room Gary was asleep and they had restrained him with cloth ties. It was to insure that he didn't get out of bed or hurt himself. As they got him ready, I called his sister and brother and other family members for support and prayers.

Chapter 5:
Praying For Intervention

It seemed like eternity until visiting hours as I sat in the ICU waiting room. Family started to trickle in as I guess word had traveled fast. Gary's cousins, uncle, aunt, his first cousin Steve, Penny his wife and her family was there from Jennings. Of course his sister Crystal and brother Terry were already there. Finally his doctor came to the door and called us in a private room to tell us what had happened.

Evidently there was built up pressure within his head, so when they withdrew spinal fluid during the lumbar puncture it allowed his brain to swell. He wasn't sure what was causing this but was keeping him sedated so he wouldn't try to get out of bed again. They were worried he would pull his IV out or hurt himself since he didn't know where he was.

That had to be a scary thing for him. It scared me that he wasn't in his right mind and nobody knew why. I was numb, confused, scared and angry. Six days and a multitude of tests and not one of them showed anything?

Surely blood tests, MRI or the CAT scan had to show something. As we went back in the ICU waiting room for visiting hours to start, I sat and cried talking to his family. Every one of them told me to get him to Houston, Texas to a better hospital with specialists and I agreed.

A MIRACLE HEALING: SURVIVING FUNGAL MENINGITIS

As I walked in the room Gary was laying there awake but not really there. His eyes were glazed over and he was motionless. It broke my heart to see my strong viral husband looking like death. I leaned over his bed to talk to him but he stared at me and looked away. He still didn't know me and I felt like someone has sucked the breath right out of me.

I held back tears as his sister came in and tried to talk to him. After a few minutes we left to let other family members come in. After his brother Terry and his cousin Ronnie came out they were both pale looking, it scared me and I asked what happened??

Gary had had another "seizure" as they called it. He went crazy again and they had to hold him down while the nurses gave him another sedative. That was it and I knew I had to make a move with or without the doctor's recommendation. I wasn't going to let my husband die.

As I walked back in a daze to the hospital room where Gary had been, I fell across on his bed and sobbed. I was so scared and lost. What was happening and why? I buried my face in his pillow and prayed. I kept asking God why and to help me, to please show me what to do.

I knew in my heart he was with us, that this was all for a reason and that somehow Gary was going to be ok. I guess I passed out for a while but I didn't sleep long and was up at 3 am praying. Finally at 5 am I made my way down to ICU to see Gary but more important to tell his doctor we were going to Houston that day.

Gary was asleep when I finally got to go in to see him and the nurses said they were trying to keep him calm so I didn't stay long. I waited in ICU waiting room until the doctor made his rounds.

As you can imagine without sleep and the trauma Gary and I had been through the previous day, I didn't mince words and went straight to the point. I told him to call the hospital in Houston and find a doctor who will take him because I was bringing him today- if I had to drive him there myself.

He asked me to wait until the results of the lumbar puncture were back but I refused saying it might be too late by then. I think he realized at that point I was dead serious and ask me to give him a couple hours to set it up.

I agreed and headed home to pack clothes for both of us. I wasn't sure how long we would be there but I knew I wasn't leaving until someone found out what was wrong and helped him.

I went home in a tailspin calling Penny to ask her if she could meet me at home to help pack. I was a mess and couldn't think straight. She was 45 minutes away but somehow managed to beat me to the trailer. She helped me pack and prayed with me and was such a blessing.

In the meantime the doctor had called to say they had scheduled an ambulance to take him to Houston in an hour. I told him I was in no condition to drive but was told I couldn't ride in the ambulance with him. I panicked at first but by God's grace, Penny had worked for the ambulance service. After a few phone calls they agreed to let me ride with him. Just another small miracle of how God puts the right people in your path to help.

We got to the hospital a few minutes before they were about to load Gary so we went to ICU. A lot of the family were there telling Gary goodbye. He was awake and talking to everyone when we walked in! I was in shock and asked the nurse what had happened. She said he had woken up a few minutes earlier coherent.

It was really strange but I think God wanted to let him see everyone before we left and say his goodbyes. It scared me in a way because I wondered if he wasn't coming home.

After they loaded him in the ambulance, I climbed in front, waved goodbye to family and we set off on the two hour drive to Houston.

Chapter 6:
The Ambulance Ride

As we began our trip to Houston in this new kind of ambulance, I was a little nervous and apprehensive. Not because the EMTs driving was bad but because they tend to go faster. Most people get out of the way when they see one coming with flashing lights. We didn't have the sirens going which was a blessing as my head was pounding with a horrible headache.

The front was cut off and short so it felt like we were riding right on the pavement. Every time someone cut in front of us and he had to brake suddenly, I felt like I was going through the windshield. I felt sorry for the driver because I was constantly grabbing the dash and holding on so tight my knuckles were white. It's comical now that I think about it but it was a harrowing experience for me.

He was really nice and even found an adapter so I could charge my phone because I had forgot my car charger at home. He talked to me a lot I guess to try and keep me calm. The paramedic was taking care of Gary in the back and I kept hearing him talking so I asked if Gary was ok.

He said yes and that Gary had been talking since we left.

I wasn't sure what was going on but I knew he was flip flopping back and forth. Although he was alert now, that could change in a heartbeat as it had several times before. I prayed God would keep him safe until we could get to a doctor who could treat him.

As we got closer to Houston the traffic got really bad and I started to have a panic attack. The EMT asked me if I was ok. I said yes but I was going to cover my face and try to relax until we got to the hospital. Driving or riding in bad traffic has always made me nervous and in the state of mind I was in, my nerves were thin and I knew it wouldn't take much to panic me.

After a few minutes we were getting off at the exit for the hospital and I could take a deep breath. I couldn't wait to get there and get Gary some badly needed help.

Chapter 7: Emergency Room Chaos

The Ambulance pulled in the hospital, unloaded Gary on the stretcher and headed inside to check him in. It was like walking into pure chaos! I don't think I had ever seen so many people in an ER. People were standing and sitting wall to wall with four admitting stations full of patients waiting to be seen. My first thought was that I was glad we came by ambulance and wouldn't have to wait. That was another disaster I was about to face.

The Paramedic and EMT went to the desk to check us in but we were told that we had to wait like everyone else. They explained Gary was a patient coming from an ICU unit but it didn't matter. I stood there with tears in my eyes in disbelief. Gary's family doctor was supposed to have set it up with a doctor here to accept him as a patient. No one told us we would have to go through ER to see him!

I was furious and scared of the thought that Gary could die right here in the ER waiting room. After a few minutes they called his name. While I stood against the wall next to his stretcher, they checked him in or so I thought.

He wasn't being brought to a room but put "in line" with the rest of the people waiting to see a doctor! The paramedic felt so bad to have to leave us but their job was through and they had to get back to Louisiana. I stood there against the wall holding Gary's hand feeling alone and scared praying for God to help us.

It was a bit unnerving as nurses and doctors were running around, screaming children, loud speakers calling people's names and so much chaos. I starting doubting what kind of hospital I had brought him to and what quality of care would he get here? Gary was moaning in pain and when I touched his face he was burning up. His hospital gown was wet with sweat and my heart pounded at the thought of waiting another minute.

I felt like I was coming apart and would scream out loud any minute when I saw a doctor walk by me. I was desperate and I grabbed his arm not knowing what he would do. I needed help and I didn't care what it took to get someone, anyone to help my husband. He spun around and our eyes met and I started spurting out everything. I don't remember exactly what I said but I know I must have left a mark on his arm from squeezing it so tight. I wasn't letting go until he helped us.

It's funny when God intervenes and lets you know that he is with you. As the doctor leaned over Gary and was doing a quick assessment, I glanced at his name on his coat. Dr. Churches. I smiled for the first time since we had arrived at ER. I knew at that moment that God was indeed there in ER with us and that he was working for us.

After asking me a couple questions, the doctor had a concerned look on his face and told me he would be right back. Relief flooded my mind hoping he would be able to get us in a room to be seen. After a couple minutes passed a nice male nurse, named Ryan, came to get us and brought us to a room. Again I smiled and thought how ironic it was because our oldest son is also Ryan and laughed at Gods sense of humor.

I thanked God as we were brought to a room hoping to see the doctor and get Gary the desperate help he needed so badly.

A nurse came in, hooked him to a blood pressure machine, took his temperature and left before I could ask any questions. After about 25 minutes I was standing at the door hoping to see a doctor on his way. Then I saw Ryan the male nurse that had brought us there earlier. I told him we still hadn't been seen and could he find out when a doctor might be coming.

He assured me he would and left. What happened next was unbelievable and it took everything in me not to call someone to take us home!

Chapter 8:
Unprofessional Behavior

After a few minutes a doctor who was seated directly across at a nurse's station walked into our room. I had noticed the nurse Ryan speaking to him a few minutes earlier so I was relieved that someone was finally going to assess Gary.

Instead of even looking at Gary's chart he proceeded to rant and fuss at me. Asking me if I wasn't satisfied with the way they handle their "business". I told him about Gary and that I was so worried about him. He told me if I didn't like the way they handled things I could find another hospital! I was shocked, hurt and angry all at the same time. How could a professional doctor that's supposed to be there helping people, seeing the emotional condition I was in and my husband laying there probably dying, talk to me like that?

I broke down crying trying to explain to him but evidently he was upset because I had ask Ryan to check on why we hadn't seen a doctor yet.

He turned around and walked out and I sank down on the chair sobbing. What had I done coming here, being treated like this, waiting in ER after coming from ICU with my husband seizing???

I picked up my phone to call family but couldn't stop crying to talk. Again I prayed to God to help us and as I finished and looked up, Dr. Churches walked by the nurses station and saw me.

He came in the room at once and I told him the whole story about Gary. It was now 10 pm and we had got to ER at 3 pm that afternoon. He smiled, hugged me and said not to worry. Within a couple minutes we were being brought to a room on the fifth floor.

Chapter 9:
A Deep Breath

As we settled in a real room I felt a sense of relief and took a deep breath for the first time since the first hospital we had entered seven days before. As the nurses came in and out doing vitals, IV's, drawing blood, a very sweet African American lady came in the room. She was an aid I guess the doctor had sent to watch Gary. He had been restrained since the previous hospital stay and they were afraid he might seize again and hurt himself.

I was glad in a way because he was so strong when he had seized the first time and I knew I couldn't handle him if it happened again.

After Gary was settled, I must have looked exhausted because the aid told me I could go downstairs to grab a bite to eat and relax.

I didn't want to leave him but I hadn't eaten all day .Although it was midnight, I was glad to take some down time so I headed downstairs. I was told the cafeteria was open but I wasn't sure what kind of food was there. Anything would be good as long as I could eat. I found some potato soup, crackers and some fruit juice, grabbed it and headed back to the room.

After I ate I curled up in a recliner with a blanket, trying to comprehend what had happened and what the next days were going to hold for my husband, myself and our future. I felt like I had been in a fog for weeks and all I wanted to do at that moment was pray and get some much needed sleep.

A MIRACLE HEALING: SURVIVING FUNGAL MENINGITIS

I drifted in and out of sleep hearing Gary moaning once in a while and turning over a lot. Around 3 am the door opened, the lights came on and in came a team of doctors. I sat up as they surrounded his bed taking his chart and in a flurry of words starting discussing all of his symptoms. Present was an infectious disease specialist, a heart doctor, a liver doctor, a kidney doctor, a lung doctor and a couple pre-med students. As one doctor would suggest something others added their opinion and specialty into the mix. I was dumbfounded and pleasantly surprised. For once in the midst of this nightmare, someone was actually making sense and acting like they wanted to find out what was wrong with my husband.

I fought back tears as I answered their questions and listened intently As they discussed a diagnosis. As this was a teaching hospital they were inquiring of each one their opinion. One of the female interns spoke up excitedly and said I think I know what this is!

I sat up as she explained why she thought it could be Fungal Meningitis. Usually meningitis presents itself with a neck stiffness among other things but Gary hadn't shown that symptom. After more discussions, they left one by one. More blood work, an EEG and a lumbar puncture was ordered. As a precaution they decided to start him on Fluconazole, an anti-fungal drug.

We spent six days in the previous hospital without a diagnosis and four hours at this one with a probable diagnosis. I was angry at myself for wasting those six days and swore I wouldn't never use a small town hospital again.

As the room cleared I laid my head down thanking the good Lord above for getting us here and for giving the doctors the knowledge to find out the problem. I drifted off to sleep crying and praying. We had hope.

Chapter 10:
Hope Shattered

It seemed like I had barely closed my eyes when I heard the aid moving around. I strained to open my eyes as she was leaving. I thanked her for being there as support for me so I was able to get a little sleep. It was six in the morning and soon nurses were scurrying in to do vitals, check his IV's and such. I hurriedly got dressed and tried to look alive although I felt drained beyond belief.

I made my way downstairs to try to get some kind of nourishment in me while the nurse were prepping him for the tests ordered for this morning. I knew it was going to be a long trying day and I was going to need every ounce of strength I could muster.

Crystal, Gary's sister called on my way back to the room to check on Gary. I told her about my horrible encounter with the rude ER doctor, the long wait in ER and finally getting into a room at 11 pm. She was upset about me being there alone and promised me she would be here that afternoon to help. I was so very glad to have family coming to help. I was so alone, frightened and thanked her for making the two hour trip.

Around 8:30 that morning two technicians from the neurology department came to do an EEG, a test used to detect abnormalities related to the electrical activity of the brain. It tracks and records brain wave patterns. As they hooked Gary up he was getting elevated so I sat by his bed trying to keep him calm.

At that moment the door opened and a lady came in from the hospital social services department. She asked me to step outside. I couldn't imagine what she wanted but I stepped in the hall with her. She was there asking me questions about the incident in the ER and about the inappropriate way I had been treated by the doctor. I was told that the hospital does not tolerate such behavior and wanted to know if I wanted to press charges.

I was shocked but impressed that it was mentioned at all much less brought to the attention of the hospital board. I had mentioned it to a nurse which in turn reported it. I told them "no" but that they needed to make sure that he didn't treat anyone like that ever again.

As we were still standing there talking, the infectious disease doctor came up to me and introduced herself. We were discussing Gary and what had happened when a nurse brought her a paper. It was the results from the lumbar puncture from the previous hospital.

The diagnosis was clear now. It was Fungal Meningitis. Fungal Meningitis is a rare disease that spreads fungus through the blood to the spinal cord. Cryptococcus, which Gary had, is thought to be acquired through inhaling soil contaminated with bird or bat droppings. So now they knew what they were treating and we could go forward with a treatment to get Gary well. All of a sudden we heard a commotion in the room and ran inside to see what was wrong.

During the EEG Gary seized, kicking and flopping around so hard that he fell off the bed. As they hurried to disconnect all the wires, they sat Gary up on the side of the bed and he began to vomit. It was a black color and looked like vile. I was terrified and as more nurses came in the room, the doctor and social worker brought me back in the hall.

I think I was screaming out loud but I don't remember for sure. . I know I was screaming on the inside and couldn't understand or believe this was happening again. It was a nightmare I couldn't seem to wake up from. It didn't seem real and I just wanted this be over.

At that moment all this was happening, a neurologist had just came out of another patient's room and the doctor called him to come. As he went in to check on Gary, she had an ominous look on her face and it worried me.

It seemed like forever although only a couple minutes had passed before the neurologist came out of Gary's room. He didn't make eye contact with me but looked at the doctor with a sad gloomy look. He shook his head, never saying a word and walked off down the hallway. I wasn't sure what just happened but I knew in my heart it wasn't good.

Chapter 11:
A Broken Vessel

As I was standing up against the wall reeling from what had just happened I don't think I comprehended the full scope of the situation. As I looked at the Doctor she calmly put her hand on my arm as if she had done this a thousand times. I felt an uneasiness in my spirit at that moment. Before she even began to speak, I felt the very breath bring sucked out of my lungs and my heart was racing so fast and loud it was pounding in my ears.

She asked me if I had children and I shook my head and stuttered two boys. She then began to tell me that Gary was a very sick young man and that I should call them and my family because she wasn't sure he would make it through that day.

I felt my legs get weak and I fell apart, sobbing uncontrollably. The social worker had never left and was still standing in the hall. She came and put her arm around me and held me up as the doctor continued.

She told me Gary had a very serious disease and though he was near death they were going to do everything in their power to save him. There was a drug they could give him that might help him to survive this but the side effects were bad.

As she explained them one by one, deafness, brain damage, loss of sight, kidney failure, all I could think of at that moment was I wanted him alive. I knew in my heart that I have "The Great Physician" and if it was his will for Gary to live then none of that was relevant. I told her to save my husband and we would deal with whatever happened later. She smiled and said ok then we will get started.

All I know is I felt lost, numb as so many thoughts were running through my mind. I was thinking of how I was going to tell my boys and everyone else. I didn't know how but as I looked at my phone to call my oldest son Ryan, it rang.

It was Melanie, Gary's first cousin and as she began to ask how he was, I blurted out that he was dying and I needed the family to come.

At first I think she was confused because I wasn't making any sense. She asked me to repeat what I had just said and then said she would call Crystal his sister and everyone for me. She assured me they would be praying and I thanked her.

The social worker stood there silent until I had finished my call and pulled myself together then she offered to take me to NICU where Gary would be. I thanked her and we headed toward the elevator. It was not surprising to me that she was there when it all came down because it was Just another instance where God showed me he was with me.

Sometimes bad things happened like the ER incident but God used it as a tool for good. She was there because of something bad but God used her for good- to bless me with a needed hug and someone to lean on in a horrible time.

Chapter 12:
My Faith Tested

Everything the next couple hours was a complete blur. It was like walking through a tunnel with a thick fog around me. As the social worker helped me on the elevator my phone rang again and it was Allan our builder. He was asking how Gary was and through the sobs I told him the situation. He got really quiet for a few seconds then asked me did I want to stop working on the house. It was framed in but he offered to give me our down payment back and said he could sell the house. It was such a sweet gesture and at first I almost said yes. As a determination rose up in my spirit I took a deep breath and said no, Gary is coming home!

He again said are you sure? I knew that was our dream home and Gary's shop we were building and I wasn't taking that away from him.

He said ok and to keep in touch and let him know what happened.

When we got to the NICU unit, Gary was already there and they were getting him settled. I went to sit in a chair in the corner. I remember asking God why this was happening and to please not take Gary from me. At that moment, the hospital Chaplin walked in, came and kneeled in front of me. Little did I know that God was about to answer me through this pastor.

I was crying so hard I could hardly talk as he began to ask me why I was so upset. Through sobs I told him what the doctor had said and that I didn't want to lose my husband.

He asked me what kind of man Gary was and if I was concerned about Gary not going to heaven.

Oh no I murmured, he is a man who loves the Lord with all his heart, serves God and is his child. Then pastor took my hand, made me look him in the eyes and asked again why are you crying? It was a sobering question and I realized I was being selfish and crying for my possible loss. A peace came over me, I calmed down then told him I just didn't want to lose him yet.

Pastor put his hand on my shoulder, said to give him to God and to trust him to do what was best for Gary. A flood of emotions and thoughts filled my mind as I was taken aback to what the doctor had said about the possible side effects. Gary wouldn't want to live like that and though losing him was unthinkable for me, living like that would be worse for Gary!

Knowing he would be with the Lord gave me peace and I stopped crying. Pastor prayed with me and I told the Lord I was giving Gary to him and whatever decision he made for him I would accept.

After we finished praying, I looked at pastor, smiled and told him I knew everything was going to be ok. It was all about surrender, trusting God with Gary and our life. Once I did, he filled my heart with peace and I knew whatever happened that God would be with me always and would never leave me.

As I sat holding Gary's hand I could hear his sister talking outside his room. I was so anxious to see her and wondered why she hadn't come in. I opened the door as the nurse was telling her that visiting hours were over. I was floored and after the day I had been through I wasn't in a mood to argue.

Trying not to fall apart I explained to the nurse that my doctor had told me to call my family because Gary might die. She had just driven 2 1/2 hours to see her brother and I was so afraid this might be the last time she would see him alive and I wasn't taking no for an answer!

I didn't want to throw at fit but at this point I was way past worrying about "getting in trouble". My family were going to see him no matter what the rules said. After a couple minutes of tension, the nurse agreed to let her in. It was a relief for the moment anyway but I knew this was going to be rough.

Crystal is a strong woman and was in the process of becoming a registered nurse but she and Gary were really close. I knew how this was going to devastate her as it had me and as much as I was scared and hurting I wanted to be there for her too.

As soon as our eyes met she broke down in tears and she threw her arms around me. I knew God was going to use our friendship and love to help get through this no matter how this heartbreaking situation ended.

She looked at her brother as tears flowed down her face, touching his face. Then as if instinct, she laid her hands on his chest and began to pray. I joined her believing that God wasn't finished with Gary yet and we were expecting a miracle!

Luke 1:37 says "For with God nothing will be impossible". And at that moment we promised we would "pray without ceasing" as the word says until Gary was healed and nothing any tests or any doctor said was going to make us waiver!

As the news of Gary's life and death situation spread through our family and his job place, calls and texts flooded my phone. I could barely talk at first but I knew I needed to let Gary's boss know. Crystal offered to call him to tell him the specifics of what the doctor had told us. As they sent an email throughout the company, people were texting offering prayers and support. We were later told that most people that knew Gary were crying. He was well liked and respected at this company he had been with 25 years. It was a blessing that the people he worked with cared so deeply about him. It really touched my heart.

Chapter 13:
A Sisters Love

In between her tears and mine I began to explain everything that had happened, what the doctors thought, tests they were doing, the multiple bags hanging and the diagnosis! It was so much to comprehend and remember. I was so upset when the doctors were explaining the situation and I guess I left a lot of blanks empty while telling Crystal.

She started asking me questions that I hadn't thought of and I felt overwhelmed. Because she was in school studying to be an RN, the nurses in the NICU were glad to answer her questions, explain the medications they were hanging and even the "why". I was really glad for her at the time because she was able to learn things as well as find out information about her brother. It took some of the anxiety out of the situation.

She literally took over helping with Gary and I was so relieved. I was an emotionally mess but as upset as she was, her nursing skills kicked in. I watched her change from a grieving sister to a professional. It was what we both needed to help us to make it through this.

The Lord knew what we both needed and sent me an "angel" one of many to come through this ordeal.

It was amazing to watch her. She wet a cloth and wiped his face and arms then wet a sponge and wiped the inside of his mouth to keep it moisturized. Things I hadn't had enough wits about me to even think of.

After about 30 minutes the nurse instructed us we had to leave until next visiting hours. So we reluctantly left, holding each other as we quietly walked down the hall.

We headed to the waiting room to wait for the rest of the family to arrive. I wasn't looking forward to facing any of them especially my boys and having to tell them their dad might die.

We sat and talked about everything and anything but what the doctors said would probably happen. It just wasn't real to either of us and I think we were so afraid if we did, the reality would set in. Neither of us could or would accept that but it seemed like it was inevitable.

Eventually our family began showing up one by one. Gary's cousin Steve and his precious wife Penny were the first to arrive. The look on their faces and red swollen eyes said it all. They were in shock and wanted to know what had happened. It broke my heart and I looked at Crystal hoping she would take over and tell them the story and thankfully she did. As more family trickled in I tried to pull myself together knowing this was going to be a rough heart breaking night not just for me but for all the family that loved and cherished Gary as much as I did.

Chapter 14:
Looking Back

As each family member made their way to the NICU waiting room, I took a deep breath and told the events of this sad day. I was mentally, emotionally and physically exhausted. As I talked to each one of them the tears rolled down my face as I saw the sadness and fear in their eyes. Everyone echoed the same sentiment of why this would happen to such a good, loving and Godly person like Gary.

It wasn't fair and everyone felt as I did that this seemed so wrong. As I listened to everyone talk about Gary, I realized that in the everyday struggles of life, I had taken for granted how blessed I was to be married to such a great person.

It's strange how as adults we get so wrapped up in living life that we lose sight of the people that we are blessed to share our lives with during this short time on earth. The bible says in (James 4:14 NLT). "How do you know what your life will be like tomorrow? Your life is like the morning fog--it's here a little while, then it's gone."

After being married 15 years and raising two sons, one a special needs child we adopted, I decided I wasn't happy. Everyone says when some people turn 40 they go off the deep end. I always said that was an excuse to be stupid until it happened to me.

I think it's a mental type of thinking that your life is wasting away. You have this obsession of wanting to do everything you never got to. It was a horrible, real feeling and I used my stressful life as an excuse to have some "me" time.

It was the worst and most regrettable mistake of my life. I lost 6 years of my life with my precious husband. Although God helped us remain friends and eventually Through counseling, lots of friends and family praying for us, we were remarried. In the midst of that turmoil I gave my life to God and now I needed him more than ever.

I knew through the work of his hands he had put us back together and I couldn't imagine only eight years later that he would let anything take Gary away from me. As I sat there listening to everyone talk about Gary I felt my heart swelling with such love for him and for a mighty God that was with us now and always would be.

Chapter 15:
An Unexpected Touch

Both my sons, Ryan and Gabe finally arrived at the hospital. I had been so worried about them driving to Houston because the weather had taken a turn for the worst. It was pouring raining and my oldest son has the tendency to drive fast regardless of the circumstances. I knew the state of mind he must be in and wanting to get here as fast as possible. I prayed protection over them the whole time and relief washed over me when I saw them step off the elevator.

As we walked to the NICU, I tried to stay calm and explain what had happened. I told them he was in a coma and things didn't look promising. I was worried especially about Gabe because of his disability. He didn't handle things like this very well.

Steve and Penny were coming out of the room and were visibly upset. They hugged me and the boys and went back to the waiting room. As we went in they both just stood by the bed looking at their dad, not knowing if this was goodbye. After a few minutes I started to feel like I was going to fall apart. I didn't want to upset the boys more so I stepped outside.

As I did my youngest sister and her ex-husband were coming down the hall. Though I wanted to stay with the boys, I felt like being emotional would cause them more grief. My sister went in and I went back to the waiting room to regroup.

A MIRACLE HEALING: SURVIVING FUNGAL MENINGITIS

As I sat there alone, I wasn't sure how all this would end but all I knew was I serve a big God and I had given Gary to him. I laid this sickness at the cross and I had to trust his judgment. I tried to prepare myself for the worst, running scenarios through my mind of how I would get through this. I trembled at the thought of Gary dying, of spending the rest of my life without him. I couldn't comprehend it and just thinking about it made it hard to breath.

I closed my eyes and prayed for intervention and little did I know that as I was, God was already answering it in Gary's room in an unlikely way.

My sister had been through so much in her young life and I felt she had given up on God. I knew she believed in him but the hurt she felt made it hard for her to serve him or trust him. I understood that because I too had been there at one time in my life. But I also knew where God had brought me from and I knew there was hope for her.

As she leaned over to lay her hands on Gary to pray for him, she felt like electricity passed through her body. I think it frightened her at first. It shook her but in that instant she knew God had touched her too. It was something that would change the rest of her life.

When she walked back into the waiting room, her face was glowing. She had the sweetest smile and put her arms around me. She then told me that Gary was going to be ok and that God wasn't finished with him yet. God had showed her that through her gesture of praying for him.

Chapter 16:
A Place to Stay

After visiting hours were over and all my family that were able to come had said their goodbyes to Gary, most of them headed back to Louisiana. Crystal, Steve, And Penny were staying overnight so we started calling around for a hotel. There was a Marriott attached to the hospital but at $200 a night, we decided to look for something not so pricey.

Everything seemed to be full but we finally found a nice hotel and checked in. We were all so exhausted and went straight to bed. No phone call from the nurse at the hospital meant God had answered prayer and Gary was still alive. We were up early and back at hospital for 8am visiting hours.

Gary was still in coma and they continued to hang new medications. Crystal made sure to ask what each one was and how it could affect this disease that was killing my husband.

Most people that contract this disease have immune deficiency disorders and their immune system is already compromised. Gary was a strong healthy man and the doctors were confused of how he could have gotten it. They questioned us numerous times and at first couldn't think of any way.

All we knew is he was perfectly healthy before this sickness devastated his body. They were also watching a heart flutter he has had all his life. This medication was so strong that he was affecting his heart and the doctors closely monitored it.

We wanted a way for him to hear God's word so we asked the nurse if we could put praise music on our cell phones so he could hear it. I was surprised when they said yes because most hospitals have rules and they were really strict here. Once against the grace of God prevailed and we put our phones on gospel music.

We laid our phones on his pillow close to his ear. Although he was in a coma, the words penetrated his spirit and we both knew he could hear it in his mind. It also gave us such a peace to be bathed in God's word constantly day and night.

The day lasted forever with no sign of life from Gary and soon it was time to leave again. All of us went to grab supper before heading back to a hotel. We went to a restaurant and saw this guy that looked like a celebrity on TV. The girls kept staring at him and after a few minutes he waved and smiled. It was a tension breaker and we all couldn't quit laughing.

It was a grim situation but we didn't really discuss it. It was good to be able to laugh for a few minutes that afternoon. Soon we would be back to the reality that a husband, brother and cousin might not make it through this night. We made it back to the hospital right as visitation started so we all went in to see Gary.

Chapter 17:
God Speaks

I truly believe with all my heart, soul and mind that God can speak to us. Sometimes He speaks in our Spirit, in our dreams, our minds or through other people. It has always been my heart's desire for God to speak to me. To audibly hear his voice, give me a word or a task to do and even just talk to me as he did Adam and Eve in the garden.

I'm sure that seems far reached to some. The word says, he spoke through a donkey and I thought if he can do that then he could talk to me. What happened next was an answered prayer because although it was through someone else, God revealed his plan to me and I heard his voice through someone unexpected.

After everyone had stepped in a few minutes and prayed for Gary, I was alone in the room while the rest stood out in the hallway. Steve and Penny had both been paramedics and crystal a nurse in training so after the neurologist checked Gary, they followed him outside to bombard him with questions.

As I sat by the bed holding his hand, I prayed as tears poured down my face. Just then the doors swung open and in strolled the sweetest little black lady. She had to be less than 4 1/2 feet tall and petite. She was elderly, maybe in her 70's pushing a gigantic echo cardio gram machine.

It struck me as odd that someone of her age and stature would be pushing a heavy machine but she wheeled it like it was light as a feather.

I was immediately drawn to her singing, yes I said singing. From the minute the doors opened that beautiful old hymn, Amazing Grace flowed out of her mouth that sounded like angels singing.

I was mesmerized and couldn't take my eyes off of her.

As she hooked Gary up to do the test, she smiled at me but never stopped singing. As I sat there wiping tears from my eyes, watching Gary's heartbeat on the monitor and listening to her sweet voice, a peace swept over me. I felt like I was floating in a dream and not understanding what was happening.

As she printed the strip from the machine, unhooked all the wires, put everything away, she suddenly stopped singing. She turned to me and said "Don't worry honey, your husband is going to be just fine. Just trust God and his word". I shook my head in agreement but I couldn't get a word to come out.

As she was walking out the door, she turned and put her hand on my shoulder and again said Gary is going to be fine. It felt like electricity went all the way from my head to my toes and I sat there stunned, almost in shock and speechless.

Seconds later Steve and Penny struck their heads in and quietly said goodbye. They were going back to the hotel. Crystal and I had rented a room at the Marriott so we could be closer to him. As soon as Crystal came in and looked at me, she ask me what was wrong. I ask, did you see her? Crystal, a little confused said who? I said that little black nurse pushing the echo machine.

Again she looked confused and said she saw a tech leaving the room with the machine but not a petite older black woman. I felt a warm feeling all over me and I knew in an instant that it was an Angel. God had sent her to tell me that Gary was going to live and that he was in control!!

As I started telling Crystal about what happened, she was as excited and thankful as I was but not surprised at all. We both know God answers prayers and gives us the desires of our hearts. God had spoken through an angel, this one heavenly. I had to trust him completely and know Gary was healed.

Chapter 18
A Time of Stretching

You never really know what you have inside you until you are pushed into a situation that is totally out of your control. It's like being thrown in a pit so Cold and dark by yourself. It's one of those times when you sink or swim, give up or pull up your boot straps and trust God to give you what you need to get through it -- A time of stretching.

Its pulling every ounce of strength, energy and faith you have inside. To face the uncertain, to fight past unbelievable obstacles knowing you are in this for the long haul. Whatever the circumstance or outcome, you tell yourself, "I can do this with Gods help.

There is a saying, "If God brings you to it, and He will bring you through it". I've always believed that sentiment and in a God that never fails me.

I'm not having saying that there weren't days that my faith didn't waiver or that I wasn't afraid. I would be lying to you if I said that was true. But each time God had sent me a word through a human "angel" or through heavenly ones. I had no doubt in my mind that he wasn't through with his supernatural "miracles" for me or for Gary.

Let me step back some years and explain why this experience was so overwhelming for me and why I was such at a loss for taking care of things. Although I've worked most of my adult life, I came to depend on Gary over the years for pretty much everything I needed in my life.

We met when I was 22 and Gary was 19, just a year out of high school. He already had a great paying job. He was a hard worker, worked out with weights on a regular basis and was very independent and mature for his age. Most guys are so immature at that age and his work ethic and ability to take care of himself impressed me.

I was in love immediately but it took me awhile to convince him I was the one for him. Things didn't work out at first and we went our separate ways. The bible says, God directs our paths and within two years we had reconnected. After dating a year, we were married.

Two children and almost 27 years of marriage, I had come to depend on him a lot. I called him my "Gary of all trades" because he could work on and fix just about anything that was broken. Over the years it saved us lots of money, time and was a blessing in our lives.

He was so intelligent though he never showed it putting on this simple country boy persona, he was smarter than most people might believe.

When computers first came on the market, he bought one knowing nothing about them. I watched him read books and literally teach himself everything he needed to know about them.

He was blessed with having total recall; remembering everything he saw, heard or read. He learned so easy although he is dyslexic but that never slowed him down from anything he wanted to learn. He never went to college but has more knowledge and skills than most people Who have a master's degree. You can imagine how much fun it was to play trivial pursuit with him!

He would get questions like, what's the capital of a foreign country and know it! He heard it or read it somewhere and always remembered everything!

Over the years he always took care of everything. He took care of the household budget and bills, fixed everything that was broke and had a good financial mind. Although we were never rich, we never had to worry a lot about finances because he always kept us above water.

Even when he was unemployed, he would get miscellaneous jobs to make ends meet. So you can imagine that when this all happen, I was all of a sudden thrown in the lion's den to take care of things I had no idea how to handle.

Chapter 19:
Pray Without Ceasing

When visiting hours were over the second night, Crystal and I headed back to the hotel room in the hospital. After ordering room service and eating a much needed meal, we showered and got ready for bed. We both wanted to be up early to get to Gary's room right when visiting hours started.

Every time my phone rang I almost jumped out of my skin, worried it was the hospital calling with bad news about Gary. I trusted God but my flesh kept rising up throwing that fear of the unknown at me.

As we set on the bed talking about Gary, the sickness and the future, I broke down crying, almost to the point of wanting to scream.

I told her I couldn't go on without him and the thought of having To made my chest hurt. He was my best friend and the love of my life, living without him was something I couldn't do. She hugged me and tried to console me although I knew in my heart that she was hurting as much as I was.

Losing a sibling hurts as much as losing a spouse as I found out this past year when I lost my younger sister to suicide. I know her heart was breaking but being the loving giving person she is, she was there for me. I can never repay her for how she helped me.

We held hands and starting to pray thanking God for Gary's life, for his salvation and all the blessings he had given us in our marriage and our lives. As we prayed, tears began to fall from both our faces, each of us asking God for our own miracle we wanted to see. She prayed that she would see her brothers' eyes open and his precious smile. I prayed to hear my husband's voice say my name and know who I was.

We both prayed for a miraculous healing in his body and mind and that all the awful things or side effects the doctors said the medication could have on his body would not come to pass.

When the doctors had first started these meds and came to hang the first bag, we prayed over all his organs, brain, hearing and anything it might affect so they would all be protected. We did this every time they hung a new bag. So we knew in our hearts God would honor our prayers. At midnight as we prayed these two requests, we were trusting God to do that very thing. The bible say to be specific when asking God for something in prayer and so we did.

We laid down in silence after that and eventually fell asleep. The morning would come quick and what the day would bring was more than we could have ever imagined.

Chapter 20:
For the Love of God

The next day was here before we knew it. The alarm I had set on my phone startled me. It seemed liked I had just laid my head down but it was already 6:30 am. I had an hour and a half to pull myself together, eat and get to NICU by eight. Both I and Crystal were exhausted and not moving very fast.

About the time we were ready to walk out the door, my phone rang. It was Steve and he sounded really strange and said we needed to get there as soon as possible! He and Penny had gotten to the hospital right at 8 and had went in to see Gary before they headed home. I got this really sick feeling in my stomach and was afraid to ask the question I knew I didn't want the answer to.

After a few seconds I took a deep breath and ask, is Gary ok? He said he is more than ok, he is awake and talking! I felt weak in my knees as I heard those words and all I could get out was Praise God!!! Our prayers had been answered and we practically ran from the hotel to NICU.

My heart was racing and it felt like it took an eternity to get there. As I pushed open the door, the first thing I heard was. Hello honey in a sweet childlike voice. Gary was sitting up in bed smiling. I fell across the bed crying and hugging him so tight not ever wanting to let go of him again!

Crystal walked to the other side of the bed and he looked at her with his big blue eyes smiled and said hey Sis! Tears ran down her cheeks as she held her brother in her arms, so relieved and happy. We had both had gotten our miracle, exactly what we had prayed for.

Steve and Penny stood there with the biggest smiles and tears in their eyes. It was one of those miraculous moments. God's faithfulness and love shone through the darkness of a coma, a deadly disease and in the midst of a hopeless diagnosis. The great physician had taken care of His child!!!

I'm not sure why the nurse had not called us when Gary had actually woke up. Maybe she thought it was too late and didn't want to disturb us but for whatever the reason she didn't. As we were asking what had happened and when he had woke up, Gary said the nurse told him she had checked on him around 11PM.

The nurses sit in a glass windowed booth so they can see each patient and with speakers in the room so they can communicate with the patient. She said all of a sudden at midnight Gary sat up in bed and said "For the Love of God!!" As she went in to check on him he was wide awake, out of the coma and asking her a million questions about where he was and why!

And if you didn't catch it, yes I said midnight, the exact time Crystal and I were praying for our miracle. Sometimes God takes time to answer our prayers and sometimes he answers right as you are praying. I looked at Crystal and we smiled at each other without saying a word. We didn't have to, we knew exactly what had happened and what a faithful loving God we serve!

For the first time in 18 days, Gary was awake, knew who I was and wasn't in pain. I knew that he wasn't out of the woods as the doctors said. I knew that from where he had been, to now, was not anything but a true miracle. No matter what happen from now on, I knew God had a plan and there was nothing Satan could do to stop it. Isaiah 54:17 says "No weapon formed again me can prosper". That means nothing can prosper, not disease or anything.

This was the second time in Gary's life that Satan had tried to take him through sickness. He had staff pneumonia when he was

1 year old that almost killed him. God had a plan for his life then just as he did now and nothing can stop that. The word says in (John 10:28) *"I give them eternal life, and they shall never perish; no one will snatch them out of my hand."*

These last three days were some of the toughest in my life. My faith was tested but as I trusted my God, he was faithful and gave me back my husband. Something I will be thankful for the rest of my life.

Chapter 21: A Different Personality

A near death experience can do so many unusual things to your mind and body. This day had been as overwhelming in the best way as my hubby was back with us although with a different personality. Let me explain. As I said earlier Gary is an intelligent, loving person and would do anything for anybody but he is also a quiet calm person.

I've hardly ever seen him upset or really mad enough to lose his temper. He's probably the most laid back person I know. Getting him to talk or to participate in a conversation was always so frustrating. He always told me that when he had something important to say then he would join in.

He was very private and it was one of the "issues" we had in our marriage. I am an outgoing people person, love visiting and have people over to play games or barbecue. If it were up to him we wouldn't have ever had friends. He liked being just us and that was great -- just not my personality.

Waking up from this coma also came a new personality that I wasn't prepared for but liked so very much. He talked in almost a childlike voice, was very outgoing, very inquisitive about everything and wouldn't stop talking. It was so funny to sit and listen and watch him. He had woke up a totally different person!

Every nurse or doctor that came in the room for whatever reason would be bombarded with questions of all kinds. Like, "where are you from", "what nationality are you" or "what languages do you speak". It was so unlike him. From an almost recluse to an outgoing bubbly happy person that was glad to be alive.

It was amazing and everyone that came to visit giggled at his sudden change. They liked the "new" Gary as much as the old one and loved his zest for life. That night my brother from Lake Charles, La and oldest sister from Baton Rouge came to visit him.

Earlier in the day the nurses had noticed that when Gary had visitors, he would get too excited. This caused his heart rate and blood pressure to elevate and it concerned them to the point that they stopped any further visitation.

I felt bad that my sister and brother had driven such a long distance and weren't able to go in. They looked through the glass of the door and waved at Gary. When he saw them he started hollering their names and waving so I went outside to tell them why they had stopped visitation.

They went to the waiting room and decided to wait until visiting hours were over so I could tell them what had happened. When I came back in the room, Gary immediately ask where they were. He got really emotionally. He asked "why won't they come in to see me? Are they afraid of me?" I thought he was going to cry.

Like I said, I'm not use to him being so emotional and it was hard for me to see him like that. After I explained to him why they couldn't come in he settled down. But he had gotten too elevated again n so they sedated him so he could rest.

After he fell asleep I headed to the waiting room to visit with my siblings and to tell them the story of God's grace and mercy. How not only had he answered our specific prayers exactly as we asked but had woken Gary up at the exact time we were praying! I know it blessed them both and they agree that he was nothing short of a true healing miracle!

They stayed an hour then headed back to Louisiana happy Gary was alive and on the road to recovery. I went back NICU to visit with my husband and to listen to his account of what happened while he was asleep.

Chapter 22: The New Journey Begins

I don't think I had been happier than I was that day. I was floating on clouds just listening to Gary's voice and kept pinching myself to make sure it was real. Everyone was so excited and I was quick to call his boss to let everyone there know Gary was awake. I know all his friends were so relieved and happy by all the cards and gifts we received the next three days.

It was overwhelming but we weren't out of the woods yet. Sunday morning they scheduled another lumbar puncture but instead of wheeling him downstairs with germs everywhere, they opted to do it right there in NICU. I was so worried about exposing him to any cold or germs someone might have. His immune system was down so low that I didn't want to take the chance.

As this morning started, the nurse was in early prepping Gary for the test. They approved me staying in the room and be able to watch but after the first stick, I got queasy and headed out in the hallway. I don't usually have a weak stomach and needles don't bother me. Gary couldn't feel it because they had numbed the site but something about seeing them sticking my husband just unnerved me.

This one was only the start of many more to come on a weekly basis. I felt so sorry for him being used like a pin cushion, being stuck constantly for blood and IV's that would "blow out". They had so many bags hanging and the doctor mentioned putting a "pic" line in.

A PIC line is a peripherally central catheter. It is inserted in the arm and then advanced proximally toward the heart through increasingly larger veins, until the tip rests in the distal superior vena cava. It is used for intravenous delivery of multiple medications. Doctors thought it would be best considering all the medications being administered. I was relieved and I know Gary was too.

The following is a list of all the medications he was receiving and why we desperately needed the pic line.

1. Folic Acid: B vitamin which helps your body produce and maintain new cells.

2. Thiamine: B1 vitamin is essential for glucose metabolism and plays a key role in nervous system function and needed for good brain function.

3. Pantoprazole: Treats gastroesophageal reflux disease.

4. Acetaminophen-(650mg): Used for fever.

5. Ondansetron (Zofran): Used for nausea.

6. Dextrose Monohydrate: A solution for fluid replenishment.

7. Apresoline (hydralazine): Is a vasodilator that works by relaxing the muscles in your blood vessels to help them widen. This lowers blood pressure and allows blood to flow through the veins and arteries.

8. Ceftriaxone-IV: An antibiotic used for treatment of bacterial infections.

9. Decahedron: Anti-inflammatory used to decrease swelling in the brain.

10. Diflucan (Fluconazole): Anti-fungal used to treat infections caused by fungus.

11. Flu Cytosine: For treatment of serious infections caused by susceptible strains of Cryptococcus.

12. Enoxaparin: Used to prevent blood clots.

So as you can see, the pic line was the only way to administer all of these medications. The fight was on to eradicate this disease and no one wanted that more than me. We had hope now nothing that happened from now forward would make my faith waver.

Chapter 23:
House Building, Long Distance

Although my thoughts were totally focused on Gary's sickness, the house building resumed as planned thanks to great friends. We met this couple through a realtor friend of ours and decided to build a house. Never in a million years did I think we would be best friends in the end or that they would be an advocate in helping us build this house without even being there.

An impossible task by any means but not when God intervenes and puts good honest people in your path as he did for this time. Although they had a family of their own in Louisiana, Trisha the builders wife made several two hours trips to Houston.

The house was just framed when we left and the only thing we had actually picked out was the countertops. There was so much to do and it wouldn't have been possible without her dedication and persistence to help us.

She brought paint chips, flooring samples, tile for the bathrooms and everything we needed to complete the house. She was reluctant to make decisions about the style of toilets, tubs, mirrors, etc. but I totally trusted her judgement

It was a lot for her undertake and I so appreciate all that she did, the sacrifices her family made. Although this was their business, she went above and beyond what anyone would have done to help us.

Another angel God had put in our path ahead of time knowing that we would need their help, knowing her willingness in her precious heart to do so. God is never shocked or surprised by anything that happens.

We emailed forms back and forth, and she sent pictures of the progress of the house weekly. She was a Godsend and just another miracle God gave us in the midst of chaos. It was going to be beautiful and I prayed Gary would be able to come home healed and whole to enjoy what he had worked so hard for. But God.

Chapter 24:
It's God or Nothing

Gary was so funny and different now, childlike in so many ways and everything made him happy. He smiled all the time and when I sat on the bed he wouldn't let go of my hand. This particular night he was almost giddy. We had a room full of company and he suddenly ask me to come closer. He had something to tell me and had to whisper it in my ear.

As I leaned closer and was about to put my ear by his mouth, he pulled me to him and kissed me the longest kiss I think we had ever had. Of course everybody laughed and commented how sweet it was. I was floored because he had always been so private about our personal life.

It was so sweet yet such different behavior for him. He was so alive and although it was different, I think I was falling in love with my husband and his new personality all over again.

After everyone finally left, he made me sit on the side of the bed because he had something to tell me. He giggled like a child with a big secret, pulled me close and whispered "I've got so much to tell you", Interested I said "ok honey, what?"

He said he had talked to God while he was in the coma. I got tears in my eyes and just hugged him. Of course I wasn't surprised at all because if God would reveal himself to anyone it would be Gary. He had always been such a faithful man of God and I've never met anyone that knows and understands the word of God like him.

He began to tell me how he was moved from room to room in heaven. Sometimes in a room, sometimes in an outdoor scene but he was always in his hospital bed with his hands restrained. I thought it odd that he would be restrained but I guess it was part of how he saw it.

He was getting frustrated as he asked over and over to see God but it seemed no one would listen to him. Almost getting to the point of anger he screamed "I WANT TO SEE GOD!"

All at once he was in a room and still in his bed. At the end of his bed there was a bright figure standing against the wall. As he started raising his head to see who it was standing there he saw someone moving into the doorway of the room. He turned to look at the doorway and saw the strangest thing!

Standing there was a man dressed in a black suit with black top hat. Gary said he looked like he was carved out of a block of Styrofoam. I know that sounds really weird but in his mind that's the only way he could describe it. The man stood there for a moment and then turned and walked away. Gary started turning his head back to the figure that was standing at the foot of the bed. At that very moment he woke up in NICU, sat straight up in his bed and spoke the words "For the love of God!" (I shared this in an earlier chapter.)

After talking to several pastors, we believe God had shown him how close to death he had come. It had come for him but Jesus was there to stop him. I don't think God is finished with what he has for Gary in this life and at that moment, he sent him back.

It scared me to think how close he was to dying but a Savior that loves us both so very much, gave us a second chance at our life together.

Although I knew it was going to be a long, hard recovery, I also knew that a loving God that I had trusted with Gary's life would be there every step of the way. Healing and strengthening him until he was fully recovered.

I'm not sure why he can't remember that part now. Maybe what he told him wasn't for this part of his life and will hopefully one day will bring it back to his memory.

A MIRACLE HEALING: SURVIVING FUNGAL MENINGITIS

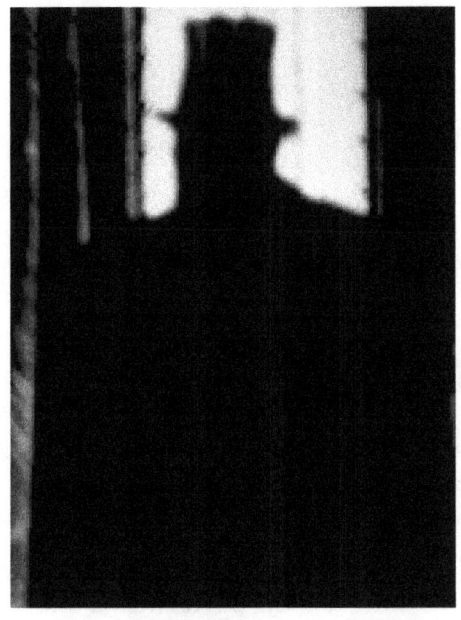

Chapter 25:
Curious Gary

With Gary's new found curiosity, everything was up for grabs. You know how a two year old ask hundreds of questions? Gary was just like that and it was comical at times. Why this and why that or what's that nurse doing, questions about everything!

A nurse came in and asked us to leave so they could freshen Gary's bed and give him a bath so it was a perfect time to go downstairs and get some fresh air.

We ended up in the gift shop, wandering around looking at everything. Crystal was across the store when I heard a squeal and then her calling my name. I hurried to see what she was so excited about and found her holding a curious George stuffed animal.

She said as she held it up. Curious Gary!! It was the perfect gift to cheer him up. She had a funny idea to put Gary's name over George on the animal. His new name would be curious Gary and she went about fixing it. She asked the lady behind the counter for scissors, tape, a black card and ink pen.

She wrote Gary on the card, cut it out to fit exactly over George and taped it. She was so excited and couldn't wait to see Gary again to give it to him. We were both tickled and it was good to be able to laugh for a change.

When we got back to the room, she hurriedly gave it to him and of course he smiled and told her he loved it hugging her. It was a precious moment I'll always remember.

Chapter 26:
Visual Distortion

Of course Gary had another funny but strange story to tell us when we got back. Ever since he had awoke from the coma, people looked and sounded strange. He said he could recognize everyone's voice -- but we all looked like sponge people. Distorted with holes and like a cardboard cut-out. I'm not sure how the swelling in his brain was affecting his vision but he wasn't seeing things very clear at all.

As he was being bathed by the nurse, he started laughing and she asked him what was so funny. He told her, "you wouldn't believe me if I told you." She laughed and said, "Sure I will."

He told her that as she would wash his arms and legs, they were disappearing!

"It's like your erasing me as your wash. I know in my mind that it's not real, but that's what I'm seeing."

I hadn't realized how much he was struggling with seeing things clearly. Later that night everyone was there to see Gary finally awake including my oldest son Ryan.

He laid there for a good ten minutes talking to Ryan but acted like he didn't know who it was for sure. I told him it was Ryan your son but he still wasn't convinced. The next thing he said was so strange and for a minute or so I thought something was wrong with him.

He asked everyone except me and Ryan to leave the room. Then he asked Ryan to stand at the end of the bed and take off his shirt. I questioned him at first and asked why? He said please just do it for me. Ryan took off his shirt and as he did Gary smiled and said. Yep that's my son and told him to get dressed.

I had totally forgotten that Ryan had a tattoo on his shoulder from being in the marine corp. Gary had remembered that and after he saw it, hugged him and was so glad to see him. It was odd but Gary's way of safely identifying him. It was so funny and everyone got a big kick out of it.

We had so many visitors that night, all relieved that he was alive, awake and praying for a quick recovery. No one was more thankful than myself to sit and watch everyone talking and laughing. Just two days earlier I had called all them to tell them he was dying. It was a miracle.

Chapter 27: The "Doctors" Diagnosis

Now that Gary was awake I thought things were looking up. I was excited to see what the doctors would say and how we would go forward from today. But the side effects of the medications were starting to affect Gary's organs. One by one the doctors came in Monday morning with their gloomy diagnosis, opinions of what they thought was happening.

The infectious disease doctor was bearer of bad news again as she told us that although Gary was awake and had made it through the coma, he was far from out of danger. The lumbar puncture had good and bad results. The medication for the meningitis was working killing the "bugs" but they were still showing positive on the culture from the spinal fluid which was causing the swelling in the brain.

Of course they knew what the medications were capable of doing to his body besides curing the fungal meningitis so all precautions were being taken and I was given the "worst " possible conclusions.

They all had their new plan of action to get Gary well and although I don't think any of them actually thought he would make it through the weekend, I could tell how happy they were and ready to go forward. Little did we realize just how long and painful this journey was going to be for my poor husband.

The following diagnosis was given for Gary two days after he woke up. Cryptococcus Meningitis, Acute Kidney failure with lesions of tubular necrosis, injury to the bladder with mention of open wound, Acute Renal failure, Disorders of magnesium metabolism, Cardiac Dysrhythmias, Premature heartbeat.

It was a little frightening to hear these things knowing that any one of them could possibly kill him or leave him disabled the rest of his life. If it wasn't for our faith and trust in God, this would have seemed completely hopeless.

Later in the morning the neurologist that had put him in NICU the morning he seized, came into Gary's room. As he picked up the chart by the bed, Gary opened his eyes and started to talk with him. The doctor was shocked as he stood there reading the chart and shaking his head. Gary asked what was wrong.

He told Gary that when he saw him Friday afternoon before leaving for the weekend. He said he had done the evaluation on him. He told Gary they have a scale they measure the brain activity by when someone goes into a coma. The scale is from one to fifteen, one being brain dead and 15 being totally normal. He had graded Gary a two that afternoon. He said to be honest I didn't expect you to live and certainly didn't expect you to be awake and talking to me.

The doctor informed him that even if someone in that condition did make it through, he wouldn't expect them to be awake or be able to communicate coherently for three to six weeks. He told Gary he couldn't explain how he was able to do that. Gary smiled and said I do, God did it he healed me. He said it was a miracle because nothing else made sense. He was one of many who would proclaim this a miracle before this was over.

Every instance of things like this happening only proved more and more that the "great physician" was in control of Gary's life.

Chapter 28: Corporate Prayer Honored

By this time the word had spread through our family and friends. Hundreds of people were praying for him, most we didn't even know. Being a child of God makes all people who love and serve the Lord our family. There were people all over Louisiana, Texas and even in Mexico praying.

I have never underestimated the power of prayer and I knew that God always honors it. Sometimes the answer is no and sometimes it's not in our time but his. Churches everywhere were bombarding heaven with prayer requests for Gary's healing.

A guy my brother worked with was so touched by Gary's predicament, although he didn't know Gary at all, prayed for him and kept in contact on a daily basis checking on his progress.

It was absolutely amazing the love, prayers, cards, phone calls and texts we received during his sickness. It gave me a new hope in people in this world. It always seemed like everyone cared about themselves and the world was becoming a cold cruel place.

This outpour of kindness and caring renewed my faith in men but more so in a God that not only answered a prayer but in doing so honored the corporate prayer of thousands of his children. By healing Gary, he not only renewed our faith but blessed thousands of his children in the process.

So many people were touched by the news of Gary coming out of the coma. Family, friends and neighbors -- everyone, everywhere -- all were touched. It was just another one of Gods ways of showing His love and compassion to one of His faithful servants.

Chapter 29:
Organ Shutdown

The joy of Gary coming out of the coma was short lived as the medication killing the meningitis was also shutting down the vital organs in his body. Although I was warned that there would be side effects of the medication, I had hoped and prayed they would be protected.

The kidney doctor came in giving the results of the most recent test on Gary's kidneys. It showed possible kidney failure and the doctor discussed putting him on dialysis the next day. I was devastated at first but then I thought to myself no!

I knew God would honor the prayers Crystal and I had prayed as we laid our hands on his organs when they hung the bags of that drug.

When I asked the doctor how soon it would be before we had to make that decision and he said the next day.

I knew I had some fervent praying to do and I knew God would hear me. I had heard so many times that once you went on dialysis you could never come off. That terrified me for Gary and I knew he wouldn't want to live like that.

As I sat on the bed next to Gary, I took his hand, closed my eyes and ask my Father in heaven to heal him. I knew in my heart he was the one who could.

Chapter 30:
Out of Immediate Danger

After five days in NICU we received the greatest news. Gary was strong enough to be moved to a room on the neurology floor. Although he wasn't out of danger (no, not by any means), he was no longer on "death watch". The medications were working but it was going to be a slow process.

I was so excited because now I would be able to stay in his room with him. Staying at the hotel running back and forth between visiting hours was taking its toll on me. I worried constantly when I wasn't there and now I could watch him 24-7. It gave me a peace in my spirit and I felt like I had more control of his care.

Within hours of getting Gary settled and all his medications flowing again, Gary was asleep resting in his own private room without restrictions of visitors. But it wasn't long before the doctors were back in checking on him and running more tests.

The kidney doctor came in to tell us that Gary's kidneys weren't anywhere close to normal but was improving enough to put off doing dialysis another day. I smiled because I knew why and nobody was going to tell me any different. God had protected them from the side effects of the medication and there would be no dialysis at all.

His liver was holding its own and the heart flutter had also calmed down. Although showed up on the heart monitor, the doctors weren't concerned as much for now. Both those things were such blessings and I knew the rest would be normal in Gods time. He had a plan and we were waiting on him knowing he had both our best interest at heart.

The 15th of April marked 20 days since the onset of symptoms this terrible disease and 12 days in two different hospitals. The journey wasn't over and only God knew when this would end but I knew now that we were going to make it to the end and that I would get my miracle!

Chapter 31: Losing Track of Time

    Healing from such an awful disease is a slow methodical process. It's not just waiting for the medication to do its job but struggling from the abuse your body has been through. Gary was so weak in his body and worn out from this sickness.

    I felt helpless as he struggled to turn over in the bed or to sit up long enough to eat his lunch. I wanted to help him but he was so independent and trying to do simple things for him made him frustrated.

    Being so strong before and now being in this weaken condition was very hard on him. Asking for help was hard and I know he felt so inadequate when I had to help him.

    The days were long and hard for both of us and I tried to hold my feelings inside. He had enough to worry about without my insecurities.

    It was really hard for me because I am an emotional person who usually Wears their feelings on their sleeve.

    I do needlework as a hobby and had brought a kit with me to work on not realizing that it would indeed be a lifesaver to me and the only thing that kept my mind busy and sane. It was a blessing and it kept me from concentrating on the long hours and days sitting watching Gary suffering and struggling to get well.

But as I said earlier I felt so blessed to actually be with him and nothing else really mattered. I knew we could get through this together.

The next shift of nurses arrived and after getting familiar with Gary's chart, they did the most unusual thing. They asked me what they could do for me! I was shocked and so very grateful. I was so lost and tired and it was nice for someone to care how I was doing.

I had a recliner in the room that reclined all the way back into an actual bed. The nurse brought me a sheet, two very warm blankets to cover with and a comfortable pillow. It was an awesome thing and I felt very blessed.

Now settled as much as you can be in a hospital setting, we were ready to face this healing journey no matter how long it would take. Gary was alive and starting to heal, we were together and God was by our side.

As I unpacked the little bit of clothes I had brought and put in a small locker in the room, I put cards friends and family had sent and a big basket of goodies the employees Gary worked with had sent.

The nurse remarked that I had it looking lived in and like home. I wanted Gary to know how much he was loved and missed by everyone. I think it helped give him the strength and determination to hang on and to get better.

It was my way of bringing home to that cold hospital room.

Chapter 32:
Quiet Down Time

With Gary settled in his private room and resting, I decided to go to the cafeteria and try to unwind. It had been a big day. Happy but tiring and I needed some quiet time. It was after the dinner rush and I knew it would be almost empty and quiet.

I went through the buffet and grabbed a couple things although I really wasn't hungry. I had not been eating much and it was starting to affect my health. The last thing I needed was to get sick also and I was already feeling run down.

As I sat at a table in the corner I was trying to hide from the few people there. I tried to take a few bites but it was hard to swallow and I felt tears swelling up in my eyes. NO! I thought to myself, don't start crying in here but it was inevitable. Tears ran down my face and before I realized it I had laid down my head sobbing.

The last three weeks hit me like a freight train and all the fear, anxiety and stress of this nightmare came flowing out like a waterfall. I looked around to see if anyone had noticed but everyone had gone. I was relieved, I hadn't planned on falling apart.

But in a way I seemed to feel better after that and releasing all those pent up emotions helped me see the situation more clearly. After a few minutes I pulled myself together and ate my meal. It was another step of healing and leaning on God. The word says "You keep track of all my sorrows. You have collected all my tears in your bottle. You have recorded each one in your book." Psalm 56:8 (NLT)

I know God was there with me, catching my tears, understanding my fears and calming me with his compassion and understanding. It was just another day in his plan for me. That gave me the strength to keep going, to lean on him.

Chapter 33: Gary Reality Check

Things seemed to be improving a little every day as far as organ function, bloodwork and symptoms of the disease. The better Gary felt the more I realized he didn't really understand the reality of what he had been through.

He was struggling with the simple things and when he starting asking about getting up I panicked. Getting up? He wasn't anywhere close to being strong enough to get out of bed must less walk. I tried not to discourage him but I was so afraid he would be devastated when he realized just how weak he really was.

Lying in bed, not eating for weeks he had not only lost weight but almost a lot of his muscle tone. My once hunk of husband with his set of "guns" and six pack tummy was thin and weak. I knew this was going to be a fight to keep him from not hurting himself in trying to do too much at first.

We got some good news the next day from the kidney doctor which told us his kidneys were functioning normal!!! Wow what an awesome miracle that was and of course no dialysis EVER!

We were so excited because he could finally get the catheter out too. He hated it so much and now it would be coming out today.

He was so happy but soon realized that it would cause another dilemma for him to deal with. Going to the bathroom was going to be another problem to face because he was too weak to walk even with a walker.

Enter the urine bottle- this was a concern of mine and it ended up being a real struggle. After being on the catheter for so long, he had trouble feeling when he had to go and when it hit, it was all at once. It was just another obstacle in the long process. I would be glad when they gave the ok to him to start trying to get up.

Him being the stubborn strong willed person that he is, well, that ended up being the thorn in his side. Although the doctors told him to take it easy and slow, he was determined to try to do things for himself.

I was glad he was feeling good enough to even try but in the back of my mind I was worried he would over stress himself and have a relapse.

It was a possibility but it didn't slow him down.

Until the day arrived that he got the ok to be able to get up, go to the restroom and possibly even shower, he kept telling me he didn't need any help.

This morning we were brought a walker, which he made a face at and said he didn't need it. I told him he was too weak to walk without assistance but that stubborn Arnold way of his wouldn't listen.

This was a battle I wasn't going to fight so when he was ready to shower, I let him sit up by himself on the side of the bed. He kept telling me he was fine as I was hovering around him watching every move.

I just smiled and let him try to get up on his own but as I already knew, his legs were weak and shaking and it wasn't but a few seconds and he was sitting back on the bed. Now that he had gotten to see for himself, I brought the walker over and he pulled himself up.

Although the restroom wasn't far from where the bed was, it took what seemed like an eternity and a struggle for him to get there. We had asked the nurse for a chair for the shower earlier and I know he was glad it was there. He barely made it to the seat and I helped him sit down.

He was shaking and exhausted and I felt so sorry for him. He realized at that moment the reality of what he had been through and the toll it had taken on his body. He now understood why the doctors and I had warned him.

By the time he showered and shaved, I didn't think I was going to be able to get him back to the bed. He was so tired and weak and every step was tiring. Finally back in bed he promised me he would take it slow.

This was going to be a struggle for both of us but God had brought us this far and nothing could stop us from the ultimate goal of going home totally well.

Chapter 34:
A New Beginning

Although Gary had a long road of therapy and healing it was like a new beginning for both of us. Another lumbar puncture revealed the meningitis bugs were still present in the spinal fluid and with that a chance of relapse. The count was lower and that was a good sign but until it was zero, he wasn't out of danger.

It was improvement and hope for the future. The doctor had informed us the time frame for this process could be as long as eight weeks. It took my breath away at the thought of 8 more weeks in the hospital. The twenty or more days already seemed like an eternity.

I wouldn't accept it and I knew that wasn't Gods plan for us. It's funny how at a time like that you panic at first and then know in your spirit that no matter what the doctors say, God has his own time frame. I knew it wouldn't be 8 weeks because only 5 days earlier Gary was supposed to die and here he was alive, talking, kidneys functioning normal as well as all his other organs, the "bugs" count was lower and he was up and walking.

God had other plans and I knew the healing was coming way before them. Even his heart rate and blood pressure were now staying normal when he had visitors. Although he still got excited, it was pure joy to see him smiling again.

The next day his cousin Melanie and her husband Robert were coming to visit. I told them beforehand about how Gary had changed and how his face was lit up all the time. It was kind of funny in a way. His voice was almost normal and he was slowly coming back around to his own personality but he was still childlike in so many ways.

I watched my words and was very careful how I handled situations that arose. He was very emotional, so opposite from before. It was an adjustment for me too. We had multiple disagreements over the years about him showing his emotions. When I was upset or hurt, I wanted him to feel the same way but he was so opposite from me. I guess it was a blessing although sometimes it didn't feel like it.

He was always the calm one and I was always the emotional mess but that's what made us so compatible. They say opposites attract and we were the perfect example of that.

So to see Gary getting so excited, talking to everyone that would listen and being so emotional to the point of getting his feelings hurt was weird and a little scary at times.

It was a good change, something I had prayed for and I would eventually get used to. It was like having a new friend and I loved it. It was strange and a new beginning to the next chapter of our lives on this journey.

Chapter 35:
Joyous News

As family and friends came to visit and saw Gary sitting up in bed laughing and talking, the joyous news of his ongoing miraculous recovery spread like wildfire. We had so many friends, family and some people we didn't even know calling and texting sending congrats and prayers.

The sadness and tears from just days before had turned into tears of joy and relief. So many cards and gifts were delivered in the next weeks and it was overwhelming to see how loved and well thought of Gary was.

He has always been a great friend and loyal co-worker who is always willing to lend a hand whenever needed. He was always available to help no questions asked and fair and honest to everyone he came in contact with.

This outpouring made me even more proud of who he was and how blessed I was to be married to him. I've always used Gary as an example when instilling in my sons the way to live and treat people. Honesty, integrity and fairness is how to treat people and that their dad portrayed all these things.

This was such a great life lesson for them to see how to live. To have such a great husband and father for my kids was a blessing in itself and with God and Gary by my side I couldn't ask for anything else.

Chapter 36:
The Nurses

Wow, where do I even began to tell you about the many nurses we were blessed with along our harrowing journey. From the first day Gary was on the fifth floor-the neurology floor, we knew we were going to well taken care of.

Every day the nurse nurse Nurse that came in would write would write their name on the bulletin board in marker. The name of the RN was written on top and the aid's name was written on the bottom. And from the first day we knew that God, with his sense of humor we loved would show us he was with us. Their names said it all. . Every week as the shifts changed, God sent us Blessings, Mercy, and Grace as nurses and it was always a mystery who we would get the next week.

One day a new RN cane in to sign her name, she was from another country. The aid had already signed her name and it was "Blessings". After she signed in Gary asked how to pronounce her name. Gary commented that we had Blessings and herself today. The RN laughed and smiled. Gary said why are you laughing? Blessings Are a good thing! She said I laughed because in my native language my name means blessings. Gary smiled and said "Look, God sent us double Blessings today!" It made his day even brighter!

The aid was there every morning and afternoon always checking making sure we had fresh linens. She always brought extra sheets and warmed blankets. She was so concerned about the uncomfortable recliner I had to sleep in.

It laid all the way back almost like a bed so it wasn't too bad and she brought extra pillows to try to make me comfortable. I know that probably seems like a trivial thing but when you are staying in a hospital for any length of time, it's hard to be anywhere close to comfortable.

Every day she asked if I needed anything after taking care of Gary's needs. It was just amazing how caring they were.

Of course doctors were in and out so much during the next week. The diagnosis was looking more promising but they never gave us false hope. We knew he wasn't out of danger by any means but every day got closer to being cured.

I was up most mornings by 6 AM dying for that first cup of coffee. A really sweet nurse would see me every morning at the nurse's station waiting for a fresh pot coffee to finish brewing. Eventually I found out where everything was and before long I was making coffee for myself and the nurses.

They were grateful because so many times they got busy and didn't have time. I got to be really good friends with all of them. One morning a new aid came in the room. She had notice me at the coffee machine numerous times.

She asked me what I took in my coffee and I told her. I wondered why she asked but so much was going on I totally forgot about it. The next morning at six am to my pleasant surprise, she came in the room carrying a cup of fresh coffee. I was floored and grateful for her thinking of me and this kind gesture.

Every day after that she was there with a smile on her face and a cup of coffee just like I liked it. It was so much more to me. She was my "coffee" angel and just another one God sent my way in a time I needed her most.

It's in the oddest situations that you make the best friends and I found one because of a cup of coffee. We talked daily sharing things about our families and our lives. She was an awesome nurse and I considered her a great friend. On her days off I felt lost, not because of the coffee deliveries but because I missed our talks.

I was there alone with no family in this town and no one to

talk to or a shoulder to cry on. She was very understanding and was a good listener. It was nice to have someone to converse with.

It was back to the nurse's station on those days looking for coffee. I'll never forget one day they were having a doctors meeting in the nurses station lounge, where the coffee pot was. I must have looked in a panic when the door was shut and the room full of people because a nurse at the station ask me what was wrong.

I told her I needed my morning coffee to be able to function. She laughed and asked me what I took in my coffee, walked into the meeting to the coffee pot, fixed me a cup and brought it out to me. I was in disbelief and hugged her. This was the attitude and sweetness of all the nurses on this floor.

My most special angel of all was an older nurse who was on the night shift. She was so attentive to Gary's needs and to mine. One day she saw my dirty clothes in a garbage bag and asked me where I was washing my clothes. I hated having to tell her because I didn't want her feeling sorry for me.

Since Gary had moved to a room, I had been renting a hotel room every Saturday just to be able to use the free laundry room associated with the hotel. Only with the room card could you get in so I was spending one hundred forty dollars a week to wash my clothes.

She had a fit and told me from now on until we went home, she was bringing my clothes home and washing them for me. Of course I told her no way but she insisted and I eventually let her. What a blessing that was to me. Every week on Friday she stopped by to pick them up and dropped them off the next morning clean and folded.

Even on the day before her day off she would still pick them up and bring back the next day even though she was off. She was my "clothes angel" and she will never understand what that awesome gesture meant to me. I will never forget her.

All the nurses during our stay were a blessing to us no matter what their names were. God had put us in the best place with the best doctors and nursing staff we had ever encountered. It was a blessing indeed!!!

Chapter 37:
1000 Questions

As time progressed I figured Gary would slowly return to his old personality but I was dead wrong. He continued to ask 1000 questions to everyone that entered the room, even the girl that came to pick up the dinner trays. When he was taken for lumbar puncture I could hear him questioning the aid all the way down the hall.

It was a conversation starter for him and he remembered everything they said .The one thing this disease hadn't taken away was his total recall ability. I was starting to grow use to the "new" Gary. He was so much like me now and that was a good thing so I thought.

My main question I asked over and over in my mind was when this nightmare was going to end. Some days I got weary and sad but God knew and always intervened when that happened.

One day in particular I had been really tired, hadn't been sleeping or eating well. The aid "Blessings" came in that morning with the biggest smile on her face. It was contagious when I saw her and couldn't help but smile back. She could tell I was down and when she was leaving, and she stopped and said "God knows your pain and it won't be long now".

I felt a warm feeling pour over me and I knew it was my wake up call. From then on no matter how bad I felt, I would recall her words and it would bring a smile to my face. It was God's way of giving me peace in the midst of this storm.

It was nearing my birthday and as it got closer I prayed to be able to go home by then. But with another positive lumbar puncture culture, it looked like that wasn't going to happen.

The day of my birthday I got the biggest surprise! Not only did the staff bring me a cake and a gift card, My sister in law Anja and brother J.R. from Louisiana came to visit. It was so great to see them again. I was so lonesome for my family and this was a pleasant surprise.

Anja, my sister in law brought me several gifts as well as Gary a few things too. We laughed about the night my brother and sister had come to NICU and couldn't go in and how Gary thought they were afraid of him because he talked funny.

He had such a childlike voice when he woke up but it was back to normal now. It was a good visit but at the end I could tell Gary was getting elevated so I told them he needed to rest. They left a few minutes later telling us they would be praying for a quick recovery.

We had another visit the next day from his brother Terry. Gary got a little emotional while he was there as did Terry. It was hard seeing his brother sick like this. Only a year earlier we had buried their mom who died from cancer and the previous year their dad. It was hard on them but we were grateful mom wasn't here. She would have made herself sick worrying about Gary.

One of those things God knew ahead of time. It was a short visit but Gary was so happy he had come by. Hopefully the next time they saw each other it would be for a Sunday dinner at home.

His first cousin Steve I mentioned earlier stopped by on his way out of town as he was traveling to a job site. Gary was so glad to see him and I think Steve was glad to see him looking like himself again.

Steve and his wife penny had been there from the start, watching him dying, praying for a miracle as we all were. They were back and forth and were such a blessing and a comfort to both Gary and myself. We are both blessed to have such great supportive families especially in times like these.

We had many others visitors the following weeks. The food and supplies they brought were such a blessing and helped so much with our finances. Eating three times a day in a cafeteria was expensive but the snacks we received helped me save a lot of money. We were so very blessed by so many people.

Chapter 38: Faith and Determination

The following days and weeks seemed endless as we went through each daily routine of test after test. The lumbar punctures were being done every 5 days and then waiting a week for the culture to grow. The day of the results were nerve racking waiting to Hear good news. But week after week the disappointment was devastating. How long could it take to kill this disease?

It was hard to understand especially when Gary seemed to be getting stronger and healthier every day. All his organs were functioning normal, he was eating like a horse and walking to the bathroom practically on his own. Yet here we were still waiting. It was hard on Gary especially because he hates hospital and being here for such a long stretch was starting to get to him.

As everything bad that was predicted that might could have happened to Gary while taking this medication hadn't happened. Blindness, hearing loss, brain damage, kidney failure, and damage to all organs. I knew it all went back to that scary day when I trusted my God and his word and put my dying husband in his loving arms. Sometimes when things seem impossible, we have to look to God and trust him in everything. Once you surrender to him, then he can step in and do the impossible in men's eyes.

I knew in my heart we just needed to hold on to Gods promises and we would see his glory revealed and our miracle come to pass. The doctors would know that the "Great Physician" was healing Gary and they would all say in the end that it was nothing but a miracle.

To make time pass I worked on my needlework project daily. It was starting to actually look like a picture and even the doctors asked to see it once a week to see my progress.

It kept my mind off the circumstances and time crawling by. It was a work in progress, kind of like Gary was.

Chapter 39: Patience is a Virtue

Pray without ceasing the word says and I did exactly that every day of our hospital stay. I know the power of prayer and not only had I seen it revealed in this situation but also so many times in my life. Not just prayers for healing and restoration but for strength and patience.

There were so many days I cried myself to sleep praying for strength to go on and patience and mercy toward Gary. Since his personality change, he was so much more emotional and irritable. Under the circumstances that would be normal for most people but not him.

He was so tired of being sick and medications to the point of total frustration. He would lash out at me bringing me to tears and it was so hard on both of us. I bit my tongue so many times holding my hurt and anger inside as not to react in the same way.

My heart broke for him and I felt so inadequate at times because no matter how hard I tried, he was just miserable. When things were calm we talked about those times and he always apologized to me. I knew he didn't mean it and couldn't imagine how he must feel.

I don't think he liked his new found emotional side either And I was worried how it would affect him mentally. I prayed for us both for strength, patient and understanding as we endured this hard journey.

I held all my emotions inside and my letting go time was always in the shower at night after he fell asleep. He worried so much about me too and I couldn't let him see me fall apart. It was one of the hardest thing I ever had to do.

I knew the time was coming that this nightmare would be over and we would look back with gratitude to a God who held us up and kept our feet firmly planted in him.

Chapter 40: Memories Lost

As the first of May was fast approaching, I thought about all the events that had passed us by that we wouldn't get back. But I also knew that we had so much more of our life yet to live, to share and to make new memories.

Easter, our anniversary and my birthday were all passed now and spent in the hospital.

I realized that it doesn't matter where you are when these occasions come around but who you spend them with that really matters. Almost a month ago my husband was given less than a day to live. Almost a month ago I was thinking about a funeral I didn't want to plan and almost a month ago I was thinking about how in the world I could live the rest of my life without my best friend, my husband.

But today as May approached I was looking ahead to spending my golden years with the man I love and almost lost. None of those events would mean anything without him with me. I felt blessed that I would get to share more Easters, birthdays and anniversaries with him. That had been my prayer from the first day and it would be until the day we were going home together.

Chapter 41: And He Walks

Gary was finally strong enough to go for a long awaited walk down the hall. He was excited as was I but as we started on our outing, it was proving be to more difficult than we realized it would be. Pushing an IV pole with multiple bags hanging was cumbersome and slow going.

I kept by his side although he was set on doing this himself. I was so worried he would fall but I soon realized he was doing just fine on his own.

It was a relief and for the first time in a month we were walking, laughing and talking and things seemed to be on the upswing. I was blessed as I watched him gliding along, smiling. He was himself for the first time since the awful headaches had started and it was amazing!

I thought at first we were going to walk around the floor but before I realized it we were headed to the elevator. I looked at him like he was crazy and asked where we were going? He just smiled and said downstairs.

I was scared at first but then I realized that if he felt strong enough then where ever he wanted to go I was game for it. We ended up in the atrium, an outside covered area with trees, waterfalls and benches to enjoy the outside.

It was so peaceful and it felt so good to breathe fresh air! We sat and talked for the first time about everything that had happened, all the mixed emotions and the sickness.

I think we made a turning point during our time there. He realized what I had been through as well as what he had. It was a relief to know he understood how I was feeling and that together we could get through to the end.

I could tell he was getting tired so I suggested we head back to the room. By the time we got back, Gary was exhausted physically but mentally he was refreshed as I was and ready to finish this journey together.

It was a really good day. Things were looking up.

Chapter 42:
A Beautiful Home Awaits

I had almost put the house building out of my mind as we struggled to get Gary well. The builder and his wife had kept in touch periodically but I hadn't realized that it was close to being finished.

I was so involved with Gary and the circumstances of his illness that the house just didn't seem important. Trisha texted one day and sent me a lot of pictures of inside and out. I couldn't believe how much had been done in such a short time. It was beautiful and I couldn't wait until we were able to see it in person.

I think they wanted it to be finished as a coming home present and they pushed the workers hard to get it finished ahead of schedule. What should have taken months was complete in 6 weeks. It was unbelievable and I was thrilled!

People say if your marriage can survive building a house then it could survive anything. Since we had left right after it was framed and now it was almost finished we never had to go through any of that stress. It was a blessing in a way. Sometimes bad things happen but God always turns them around for good. This was just another instant of his mercy and grace and I'm so very thankful!

It was nice to know what awaited us in the future but for now my concentration was totally on hearing the infectious doctor tell us the lumbar puncture was negative. That would be the turning point, the miracle that we had been praying for and waiting on for over six weeks.

Then we could go forward and plan our future in our new home. All I could think have or hope for and it WAS going to happen.

I continued my needle project in hopes of finishing it by the time we were able to come home. Sitting for all these days, eating three meals a day was taking its toll on my weight. Before the onset of Gary's headache I had been walking 4 miles a day and starting to get in shape. I felt like a big blob which added to my stress of sitting 12 hours every day.

The only exercise I got was walking back and forth to the cafeteria to get food. I was gaining weight and getting lazy and it's scared me. My mother was obese when she died at age 55 and I was always concerned when I gained the smallest amount of weight. That fear stayed with me I prayed we would be home soon.

Satan used things like this to try to attack my faith and make me afraid and that God had left me. But I knew what was happening and I didn't let him destroy my faith in a God that had brought us from sure death to a miracle healing. My needle work project completed and framed.

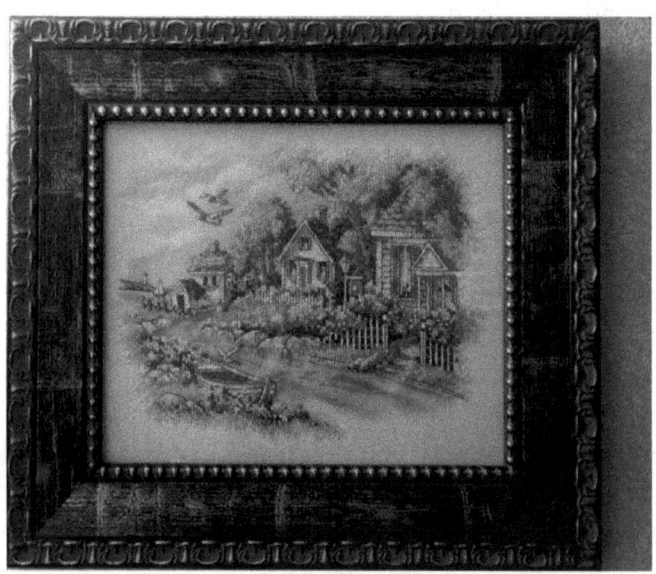

Chapter 43:
The Final Lumbar Puncture

By now we had lost count of how many actual lumbar punctures Gary had been through since he entered the first hospital. Although it was only once a week, I know to Gary it seemed like every couple days.

We were praying that the medication was finally to the point of killing the fungal meningitis and that this would be the last one he would ever have to endure.

We didn't want to get our hopes up once again only to be disappointed. It usually took a week to get the results and as we waited for the doctor to come in that day I felt in my spirit that somehow this day would be different.

I felt a peace I hadn't felt before and although the anticipation of waiting to hear was in the back of my mind, I knew today was our day for a promised miracle!

As the door opened, the look on her face said it all! She looked like she was bursting at the seams to tell us the news as if it was her own family! Something we had been waiting to hear for over six weeks, the culture showed no growth for the first time in 4 weeks!

I can't tell you the overwhelming joy that flooded my heart and soul. Gary was smiling ear to ear and his first question was of course, when can we go home? I was thinking the same thing but I knew it wasn't that simple or quick.

She wasn't ready to give us a discharge date just yet. She was cautious and I could totally understand why. Gary had been close to death and she wasn't taking any chances!

She told us they would continue to monitor him and that she wanted To get one more clear lumbar puncture before she would consider discharging us.

As much as we wanted to be out of that hospital, we also wanted Gary to be total healed and out of danger of a reoccurrence. We reluctantly agreed knowing that we were counting days now instead of weeks and that was good enough for now.

Chapter 44: Our New Goal- Home

As we waited for another week to pass in anticipation of a second lumbar puncture with no growth, we continued to pray and believe God for it. It was all in his time and we tried to be patient as we waited on him.

The "big day" finally came and hearing those words. "Another one clear with no growth" was the happiest sound we had ever heard. It was official, the meningitis "bugs" were dead. Tears rolled down my face as I tried to contain my excitement.

Our faithful loving Father had kept his promise And answered our prayers. Doctors were amazed at how quick Gary had recovered and how none of the side effects associated with this medication had touched Gary at all.

Not one of them could say anything except it was a miracle! Yes and the miracle worker himself walked by our side through the entire ordeal, protecting Gary from all the bad things that were "suppose" to happen. We had the Great Physician as our doctor and nothing is impossible when he is in control!

The other thing I had been praying about was to be home for Mother's day to spend with my kids and Gary as a family. What a great surprise that would be for the boys!

Our next question for the doctor was when can we go home? She told us he had to go to rehab and we would see. My heart fell as I listened to her explain but I knew that God would answer that prayer too. I just had to be patient a little longer and trust him.

After three days in rehab the doctor came to check on us and see how Gary was doing. After checking his chart, the doctor turned to us and said. How would you two like to go home?

We both shouted yes before she could barely finish her sentence. She laughed and said ok and then gave us all the precautions to take and what medication Gary would continue to take after we returned home.

It would be maintenance drugs for three more months to make sure the meningitis didn't come back. That was fine with us as long as we could go home. It was the Friday before mother's day in the afternoon so the doctor said the papers would be ready in the morning for us to leave.

Again I cried like a baby but this time it was overwhelming tears of joy. Gary was smiling so big I thought his face would crack. We thanked her for everything she had done and for caring so much for Gary's life. We were blessed to have her as a doctor.

Trisha, the builders' wife had called that afternoon and when she learned of the great news, she offered to come get us. It was a blessing and she made plans to be there early sat morning.

I can't explain the happiness we were feeling or the excitement of finally being able to go home.

Neither of us slept much that night and we were up and packed early. Of course it took until after lunch for the staff to get the papers ready.

Trisha was there and helped me get Gary to the car and all my luggage loaded. It was a beautiful sunny day as we drove the two hours back to Louisiana and I was so relieved we were really going home.

On the way home Trisha told us that the house wasn't quiet finished but offered for us to stay at their house until we could move into the house. That was a sweet gesture and we gracefully accepted.

They lived right across the street from where we were building so it was easy to walk over to watch the finishing touches on it. It was just another miracle God had given us. A new home and another chance for our lives.

Chapter 45:
Angels Among Us

Do you believe in angels? I was always told when I Was growing up that I had a guardian angel watching over me. It was comforting to know that although I couldn't see "her". So many times in my life I have witnessed miraculous things and I know for a fact there are indeed angels here on earth.

Some are heavenly and some are plain human beings whom the Good Lord has sent my way. In a time when I needed one most, He was always faithful to send one.

Our journey of Gary's sickness was no different. Although there was so many "angels" that helped us, there were 10 special ones I will never be able to thank enough or ever forget.

My first "Prayer Warrior" angel was Penny whom from the start until the very end was my lifeline. She will never know just how thankful I am and how I would have never made it through without her.

My second "Doctor Angel" was Dr. Churches. Without him I would have lost my mind that day in the ER and I am so thankful for his caring spirit. He cared when no one else seemed too. I am forever grateful.

My third "specialist angel" was Dr. Drews. Her caring and not giving up personality gave me hope in a bleak situation. She never gave up on getting Gary well and she will always be in my heart.

My fourth "pastor angel" was the on-call chaplain that prayed with me that horrible day and gave me peace. He genuinely cared and gave me the best advice I would ever get in my life. He'll never know how he changed things by his kind words.

My fifth "sister angel" was Crystal Gary's sister. Her unwavering spirit and love for The Lord helped me through one of the worst times in my life. She wasn't just a sister in law but my best friend and the best help anyone could ask for. I am so very blessed I can call her my family.

My sixth "electric angel" was my younger sister Lisa. Through praying for Gary, was touched by God and gave me a message of hope.

My seventh "amazing grace" angel was indeed the heavenly kind that God sent to comfort and reassure me. She touched my very soul with her song and words that only came from God. She let me know God was right there with us.

My eighth "house angel" was Trisha. Without her determination, thoughtfulness and sacrifice, we would have never got our house built. She went out of her way to help get that accomplished and I am forever in her debt.

My ninth "coffee angel" was a sweet young black nurse that took time out of her busy schedule to bring me coffee every morning. We became good friends and she touched my heart with her kindness.

My tenth and final angel was my "clothes angel". Through her kind act of washing my clothes weekly, she saved me hundreds of dollars in hotel room rentals. But more than that she gave me a renewed hope in people.

I was truly blessed by all of these and so many more and I can never express how thankful I am.

Chapter 46:
Moving Day

The doctors had warned Gary to take it easy for a while. His body and brain had been through a lot of trauma and we were worried he would relapse if he did too much. Stubborn as he was I knew it would be a struggle to keep him from doing too much.

Although he was well, his strength was limited and after a couple days of doing minor things brought him to the realty that he wasn't the person he was before he got sick.

It was frustrating for him and made him angry at himself. When moving day was finally upon us, I made sure we had adequate help to move everything without Gary having to do too much. Several times I had to almost get ugly with him to make him rest.

It was June in Louisiana with the temperatures in the 90's and the heat took its toll on him within a short time. Once we got everything loaded out of storage and to the house, we let everyone go home because the builder offered for his crew to unload the trailer.

That was a big blessing and saved him from doing more than he should have.

I wasted no time getting things unpacked and organized as fast as possible. After the ordeal we had been through I just wanted some kind of normal in our lives again.

It was so nice to be home and settled and ready to share the next part of our journey God had for us. I don't think I realized the little things that had been affected by this disease.

Gary was having some short term memory issues and simple things like measuring things frustrated him. He had always been a math whiz and could figure out measurements and solutions in his head without paper or pencil.

Other things I noticed in the first couple weeks was how forgetful he was. I would tell him things and later he wouldn't remember and swear I didn't tell him. It started to concern me.

After a couple more things happening I called the doctor one day to explain what was going on. She wasn't concerned and told me sometimes cognitive abilities are slightly off for a while until the brain "reboots" itself. I was relieved and from that point on tried to reassure him it was temporary.

Within weeks he as back to his old self, growing stronger every day and getting into working in the yard. It was good to see him happy again.

Chapter 47: What Really Matters

We finally got the house in order and Gary wanted to start working on the yard and building his shop in the back. He took it slow and it really seemed to help his spirits and also mentally and physically.

With three months he was talking about going back to work. I thought it was a great idea so we called the doctor to get her opinion and see when he would be finished with the medications.

She totally approved so the next day he called his boss and informed him he would be back.

It seemed like everything was falling back into place and things were going to settle down. But I noticed something that was concerning me and I thought I might need to take a second look at our situation.

After a day of simply moving the yard on a riding lawn mower, he would be exhausted. Being in the heat doing anything wore him out and it always took a couple days to feel strong again. I was beginning to wonder if this big house and yard and building that shop was going to be too much for him.

After a trip that next week to the doctor for a checkup and getting the all clear, it was a day of celebration, no more medication and no more follow up visits. We were totally done with all that and it was the best news!

The next couple weeks we discussed so many things about the past, the illness and our future. We had a beautiful home, something we dreamed about, sacrificed for and struggled to save for. It was finally accomplished and real.

It is funny how something that seems so important and you work so hard for so long, doesn't seem so important once you have it.

Once you go through a trial in your life where you almost lose someone important in your life, your priorities change. After the first of the year we sat down one day and had a long revealing talk, and found out we had been feeling the same way.

We wanted to be out of debt and be able to enjoy our life together and this house just wasn't important to either one of us. We decided to put it on the market after a lot of serious praying. I guess it was what the Lord wanted.

We had listed it fully furnished as we had bought all new furniture. We planned on buying an RV and eventually traveling when Gary retired. Within 3 days of listing it a young couple came to look at it, bought it furniture and all. That just doesn't happen and we knew Gods hand was on the sell and we had made the right decision.

Once again God had answered our prayers and granted us yet another miracle.

Chapter 48:
The Rest of the Story

Within two weeks we had closed on the house, bought an RV and moved in a nice RV park. I thought our life would finally settle down and be simple. But Gary had other ideas and I was shocked when he came home one Friday with some unusual news!

He told me he had taken vacation the next week and we were going to Alaska! I was stunned and excited at the same time. It had always been on our bucket list to visit Alaska but I really never thought we would ever get to go.

I was in a panic to get airline tickets, find a place to rent and get a rent car in three days. I met a sweet lady on a travel site and she ended up taking care of all of it for me. The following Monday we were headed to Sitka, Alaska. It was a dream come true!

I fell in love with Sitka and I cried the day we left to come home. I knew I had found my place of peace. I also knew it was just a dream to be able to live there.

The bible says God gives you the desires of your heart and I knew he was seeing mine. After we got home we talked intensely about it and one year later, we had sold our RV, Gary had retired and we were headed to Alaska.

God blessed us with a beautiful condo right on the Pacific Ocean where we can sit on our porch watching sea otters, sea lions and whales not to mention eagles.

It's our miracle healing of our hearts and a reward for trusting a faithful loving God, who brought my husband from sure death to a healthy thriving man and changed what could have been crippling for me into a true miracle. He gave me back my husband and my life and I will forever love him and praise him!

For anyone who is facing a battle from disease, financial trouble or any situation that seems hopeless, look up! We serve a merciful loving faithful God who loves us so very much that he sent his son to die for us and our sins.

He knows what you are going through and what lies ahead. He will be there with you every step of the way. So please don't give up, your miracle might be just around the corner. Trust him, he will never leave you or forsake you. He still works miracles every day! We are living proof there is a God in heaven and he rules and reigns forever!!

Healing Scriptures

"BLESS the LORD, O my soul; And all that is within me, bless His holy name! Bless the LORD, O my soul, and forget not all His benefits. Who forgives all your iniquities, who heals all your diseases?" (Psalms 103:1-3 ESV).

"Many are the afflictions of the righteous, but the LORD delivers him out of them all." (Psalms 34:19 ESV).

"Then they cried out to the LORD in their trouble, and He saved them out of their distresses. He sent his word, and healed them, and delivered them from their destructions." (Psalms 107:20 ESV).

"Beloved, I pray that you may prosper in all things and be in health, just as your soul prospers." (3 John 2 ESV).

"Then your light shall break forth like the morning, your healing shall spring forth speedily. And your righteousness shall go before you, the glory of the LORD shall be your rear guard." (Isaiah 58:8 EVS).

Faith Scriptures

"So faith comes from hearing, and hearing through the word of Christ." (Romans 10:17 ESV).

"And without faith it is impossible to please him, for whoever would draw near to God must believe that he exists and that he rewards those who seek him." (Hebrews 11:6 ESV).

"And Jesus answered them, "Have faith in God. Truly, I say to you, whoever says to this mountain, 'Be taken up and thrown into the sea,' and does not doubt in his heart, but believes that what he says will come to pass, it will be done for him. Therefore I tell you, whatever you ask in prayer, believe that you have received it, and it will be yours." (Mark 11:22-24 ESV).

"For nothing will be impossible with God." (Luke 1:37 ESV).

"Now faith is the assurance of things hoped for, the conviction of things not seen." (Hebrews 11:1 ESV).

Hope Scriptures

"Rejoice in hope, be patient in tribulation, be constant in prayer." (Romans 12:12 ESV).

"For I know the plans I have for you, declares the Lord, plans for welfare and not for evil, to give you a future and a hope." (Jeremiah 29:11 ESV).

"May the God of hope fill you with all joy and peace in believing, so that by the power of the Holy Spirit you may abound in hope?" (Romans 15:13 ESV).

"Be strong and courageous. Do not fear or be in dread of them, for it is the Lord your God who goes with you. He will not leave you or forsake you." (Deuteronomy 31:6 ESV).

"But they who wait for the Lord shall renew their strength; they shall mount up with wings like eagles; they shall run and not be weary; they shall walk and not faint." (Isaiah 40:31 ESV).

"Then your light shall break forth like the morning, your healing shall spring forth speedily. And your righteousness shall go before you, the glory of the LORD shall be your rear guard." (Isaiah 58:8 ESV).

"Then they cried out to the LORD in their trouble, and He saved them out of their distresses. He sent his word, and healed them, and delivered them from their dust." (Psalms 107:20 ESV).

Love Scriptures

"So that Christ may dwell in your hearts through faith—that you, being rooted and grounded in love, may have strength to comprehend with all the saints what is the breadth and length and height and depth, and to know the love of Christ that surpasses knowledge, that you may be filled with all the fullness of God." (Ephesians 3:17-19 ESV).

"For I am sure that neither death nor life, nor angels nor rulers, nor things present nor things to come, nor powers, nor height nor depth, nor anything else in all creation, will be able to separate us from the love of God in Christ Jesus our Lord." (Romans 8:38-39 ESV)

"So we have come to know and to believe the love that God has for us. God is love, and whoever abides in love abides in God, and God abides in him." (1 John 4:16 ESV).

"No, in all these things we are more than conquerors through him who loved us. For I am sure that neither death nor life, nor angels nor rulers, nor things present nor things to come, nor powers, nor height nor depth, nor anything else in all creation, will be able to separate us from the love of God in Christ Jesus our Lord." (Romans 8:37-39 ESV).

"Why, even the hairs of your head are all numbered. Fear not; you are of more value than many sparrows." (Luke 12:7 ESV).

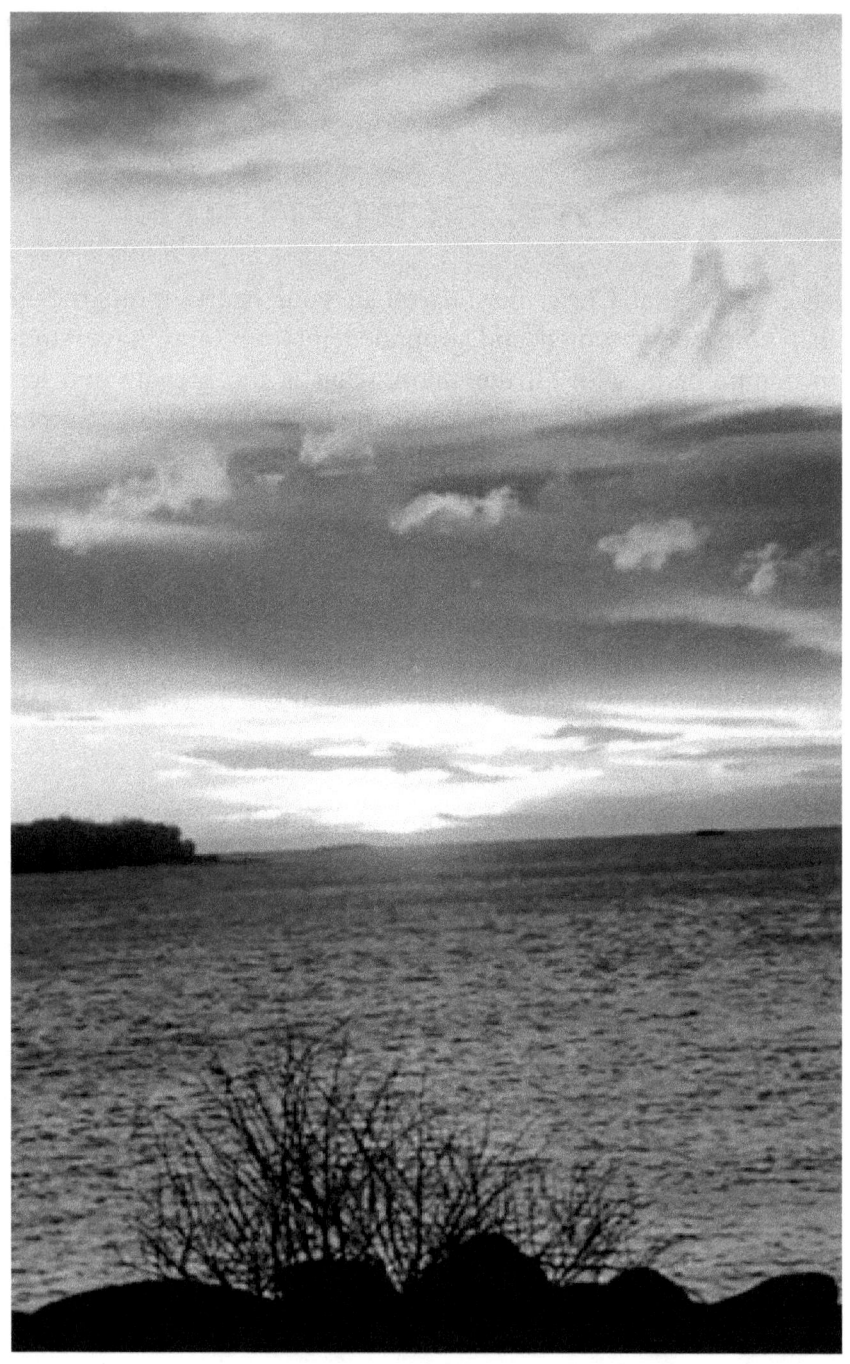

SUNSET FROM OUR HOME
SITKA, ALASKA

Judy Arnold

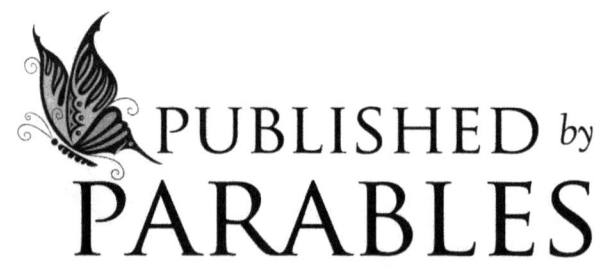
Earthly Stories with a Heavenly Meaning

www.ingramcontent.com/pod-product-compliance
Lightning Source LLC
Chambersburg PA
CBHW071718020426
42333CB00017B/2320